THE WISDOM
OF CRYSTALS

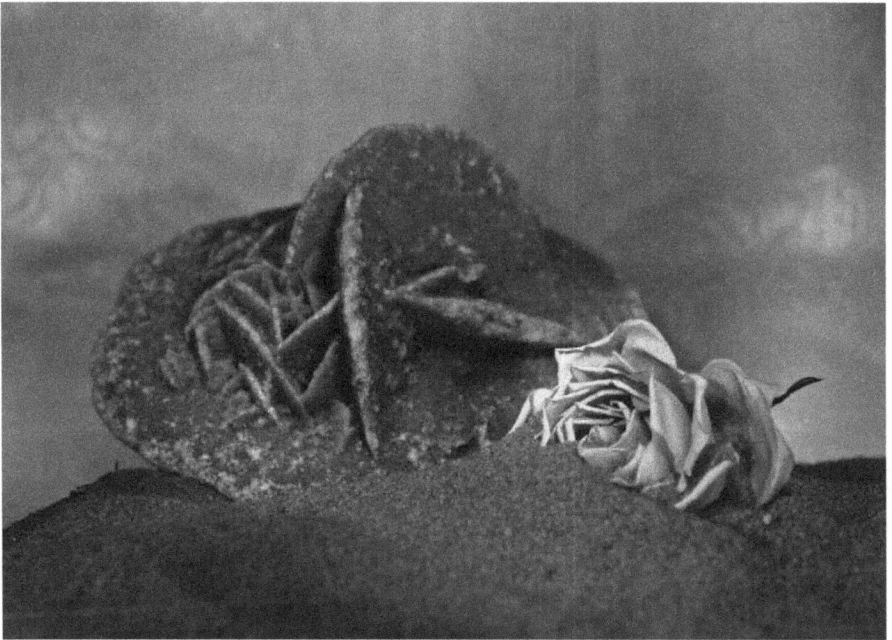

MICHELE DOUCETTE

The Wisdom of Crystals

ISBN 978-1-935786-05-4

Printed in the United States of America by

St. Clair Publications

PO Box 726

McMinnville, TN   37111-0726

http://stanstclair.net

Acknowledgments

I wish to thank Luis Garcia Marín, from Torremolinos, Malaga, Spain, for permission to use his *Hombre de cristal* (Crystal man) photograph (cover image) as well as his *Rosa del desierto* (Desert Rose) photograph (inside cover image).

A graphic designer as well as a photographer, you can visit his personal webpage at http://www.luimalaga.com/ as well as his alluring and intriguing online Flickr album at http://www.flickr.com/photos/luigmarin/

Gabriele Lanoue, co-owner and proprietor of The Inner Peace Awareness Center [1] in Saskatchewan, Canada, was my Stonebridge College tutor. It was a privilege to be able to work with her, obtaining my Crystal Healing Practitioner diploma in 2005.

I wish to thank Kellie Jo Conn, the Crystal Deva, [2] for working with me on this project. In the chapter pertaining to crystal formations, you shall be greeted with visual images of beautiful crystal beings.

---

[1] http://www.innerpeaceawareness.com/
[2] http://www.avaloncrystals.com/

In addition, the names that follow are the *key reputable sellers* of crystals that I have purchased from over the years.

Barbara Yvette Allen, known to eBayers as Crystalmoon. [3]

Barbara Babel, known to eBayers as Crystalline Rainbows. [4]

Debbie Frank and Grace Mattson, known to eBayers as Gemfinders International. [5]

Joe George, known to eBayers as Cascade Scepters Mineral Specimens. [6]

Annie Goldman, known to eBayers as Jewel Wraptures. [7]

Robyn Harton, owner and proprietor of Robyn A. Harton Creative. [8]

Bonnie Langley, known to eBayers as Bonnies Crystals. [9]

Eleanor McDonnell, known to eBayers as Moon in Aquarius. [10]

---

[3] http://stores.shop.ebay.ca/Crystal-Moon-Jewelry-Designs
[4] http://stores.ebay.ca/Crystalline-Rainbows
[5] http://stores.shop.ebay.ca/Gemfinders-International
[6] http://stores.shop.ebay.ca/Cascade-Scepters-mineral-specimens
[7] http://stores.ebay.ca/Jewel-Wraptures
[8] http://www.crystalsandjewelry.com/
[9] http://stores.shop.ebay.ca/BONNIES-CRYSTALS

Maeve Ross-McKee, known to eBayers as Betty's Bodacious Beads and Gifts. [11]

Sherry Whitfield Merrell, known to eBayers as Blue Star Traders [12] (and owner of the ancient crystal skull, Synergy).

Genn Waite, owner and proprietor of Arkansas Crystal Works. [13]

Ken Wells, known to eBayers as Kismet Anwvyn [14] (seller of *absolutely outstanding* Moldavite).

Ravenia Youngman, known to eBayers as Crystal Skull Head Quarters. [15]

To my husband, Albert Stewart, who steadily encourages me to write. After twenty-five years, he continues to remain my confidant, my anchor, my closest companion.

To my children, Alyssa and Niall, may they also continue to learn more about themselves in association with their guardianship of many mineral kingdom companions.

---

[10] http://stores.ebay.ca/Moon-in-Aquarius
[11] http://stores.shop.ebay.ca/Bettys-Bodacious-Beads-and-Gifts
[12] http://stores.shop.ebay.ca/Blue-Star-Traders
[13] http://www.arkansascrystalworks.com/
[14] http://stores.ebay.ca/Kismet-Anwvyn
[15] http://stores.shop.ebay.ca/Crystal-Skull-Head-Quarters

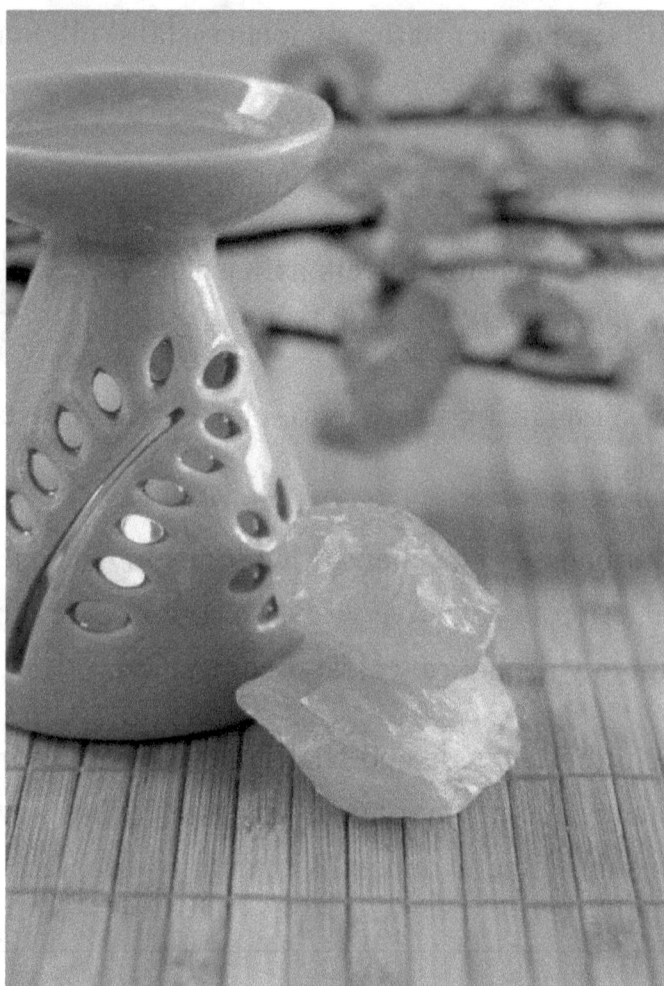

Table of Contents

Disclaimer 1

Reviews 2

Introduction 5

Frequencies... 8

Crystal Insights 11

My Final Exam 15

Hand Brushing...25

Choosing Your Crystals......................................27

Cleansing of Crystals 29

Facilitators of Healing....................................32

Ready to Begin 33

Exploring Your Crystals 35

Crystal Energy Exploration Techniques 46

Crystal Visualization Exercises.............................49

Directory of Crystals.......................................51

Pendulum Dowsing..68

Getting To Know Your Pendulum 71

Crystal Formations..75

Beliefs about Quartz Crystal 120

The Subtle Energy of Crystals and Stones.........................123

Quartz Crystals with Special Properties 130

Structured Water, Quartz and Your Health 150

The Chakras...154

Crystal Layouts...161

Book Source Bibliography...164

Internet Source Bibliography 166

Favorite Crystal Websites 167

Accredited Crystal Healing Courses 169

About the Author 171

Disclaimer

All information and material located within this publication is provided for general informational purposes only.

While unsubstantiated from a scientific perspective, all metaphysical healing lore discussed within these pages has been provided for

[1] inspiration,

[2] folklore, and

[3] entertainment purposes only.

In making use of this publication, the reader both acknowledges, and agrees, that they must assume complete responsibility for their use and/or misuse of this information.

We must continue to realize that we are healing facilitators and not healers.

Michele, what I *really* like about your book is that it is *more of a crystal healing course*, one that is wonderful.

I like how you encourage the reader to write down everything they are feeling and sensing. That is brilliant.

I am *so glad to see that you do not recommend clearing in salt* of any kind, an old school method that is *actually harmful*.

I like how you explain both color, and lack of, under your Directory of Crystals chapter; kudos to you.

I feel that your book is *so appropriate* for the *beginner crystal healers* out there. I know many who are just starting out and need help to learn. Your book would be *the perfect accompaniment* to their learning.

Kellie Jo Conn, Avalon Crystals, The Crystal Deva

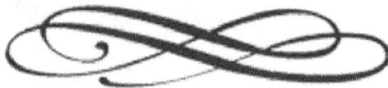

A great read for anyone who loves crystals, from beginners to those who have been working with crystals for a long time.

Michele has done a wonderful job in creating a *comprehensive guide* in an easy to read and understand format. I will definitely be adding this book to my crystal library!

Kristi Huggins, author of *Gemstone Healing Guide, A Healing Apothecary* and *Stepping Stones to Crystal Basics: Crystal Communications Course*

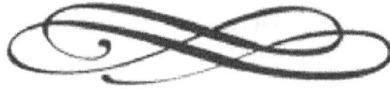

A *very well written book*, ideal for anyone who wishes to understand more about stones and crystals and how to best connect with and care for them.

Michele Doucette's style of writing and presentation are very easy to follow and understand. I highly recommend this *wonderful guide* to anyone who wishes to further their knowledge in this fascinating field.

Ravenia Youngman, Crystal Skull Head Quarters

Michele's explanation of high and low level frequency and illness/healing is very interesting. The reader is certain to find lots of information on crystals, gemstones, chakras and even crystal layouts and meditation. I believe *there is plenty in this book for everyone*, beginners as well as advanced crystal practitioners.

As always, Michele's writing is *interesting, concise* and *informative*. She includes many exercises and instructions for a person to get to know their crystals on a more intimate level.

I recommend this book for anyone wanting to become more familiar with themselves and how to work with their crystal friends.

Genn Waite, Arkansas Crystal Works

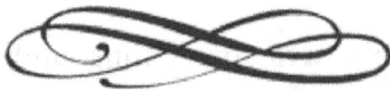

Piezoelectricity is the ability of some materials to generate an electric potential in response to applied mechanical stress. There are many materials, both natural and man-made, that exhibit this piezoelectric effect. In keeping with crystals, the topic of this book, there are several that demonstrate this piezoelectric effect – Quartz, Berlinite (a rare phosphate mineral that is structurally identical to Quartz), Topaz and minerals from the Tourmaline group.

Direct piezoelectricity from Quartz can generate thousands of volts. That having been said, modern science already harnesses the power of crystals in everyday life as has been evidenced by radio, television and satellite communications. Both computer technology and laser surgery make use of the electromagnetic energy of crystals.

The catastrophic downfall of Atlantis has been attributed to the very misuse of this piezoelectric energy. Although first written about by Plato some 2,500 years ago, such continues to hold steadfast appeal in that scientists, historians, archaeologists and geologists have now entered into the debate, all trying to contest the various literary, historical and geographical elements of the story.

The Wisdom of Crystals

Edgar Cayce first made mention of Atlantis in a life reading given in 1923. He was later to give its geographical location as the Caribbean. In addition, he further proposed that Atlantis was an ancient, highly evolved civilization, complete with ships and aircraft powered by crystal energy.

While others equate the sudden downfall of Atlantis with the sudden downfall of the Minoan civilization, the volcanic eruption at Thera, around 1,500 BCE, does not match the time period attributed to Atlantis.

Quartz, in its many varieties, formed by silicone and oxygen (together making silicone dioxide), constitutes about 75 percent of the outer planetary shell. Other precious stones and metals occur in much lower quantities than this.

Quartz is a medium through which we can amplify energies. In addition, because it vibrates at a constant frequency, it is used in many electronic devices, including computer chips.

Although colorless in its purest form, Quartz can be transformed into almost any color by the presence of impurities that may lodge within the crystal. Amethyst, Rose Quartz, Smoky Quartz, Morion and Citrine are all different colored variations of the colorless quartz.

One of the reasons why Quartz is so effective is that its matrix is made up of tetrahedrons. Tetrahedrons are composed of four triangles together, forming a pyramidal shape (a three-sided pyramid on a triangular base). Countless numbers of these shapes are then closely packed together in a very precise way, in order to form the matrix of the crystal. As we all know, pyramids are great amplifiers of energy.

Quartz crystals take in energy through the base. Amplified through their bodies, it is then transferred out through their terminations.

Since ancient times, Quartz has been accorded mystical powers. Many people today make use of Quartz crystals as a metaphysical healing tool. In order to fully appreciate the value of working with crystals in this manner, it becomes important to understand that much of our world is basically crystalline, both in structure and substance.

The human body is also crystalline in nature. The largest single element in the human body is water, which is a form of liquid crystal. The blood is also liquid crystal. Trace minerals are all crystalline in nature. By using quartz crystals when working on the human body, it is possible to reprogram the crystalline nature of the physical vehicle.

In layman's terms, frequency pertains to how often an electromagnetic wave repeats itself. The faster the repetition, the higher the frequency.

Everything has a frequency, including color, light, essential oils, Bach flower remedies, crystals, plants, animals. You get the picture.

A healthy human body has a frequency that ranges from 62 to 78 MHz, while disease begins at 58 MHz.

Dr. Royal R. Rife found that every disease has a frequency. In continuation, he was able to determine that certain frequencies can [1] prevent and eradicate the development of a disease while others [2] are able to destroy them. In summation, substances of a higher frequency will destroy diseases of a lower frequency.

Bruce Taino of Taino Technology, an independent division of Eastern State University in Cheny, Washington, was the creator of the first frequency monitor.

This frequency monitor, built in 1992 and certified as being 100% accurate, has also been utilized to measure the influence of thought on the human body.

It should not come as a complete surprise to learn that negative thoughts lowered the measured frequency by 12 MHz while positive thoughts raised the frequency by 10 MHz. It was also found that prayer and meditation increased the frequency by 15 MHz.

Dr. Gary Young, a renowned researcher in the field of therapeutic essential oils and founder of Young Living Essential Oils, Inc., discovered that if the frequency of the left and right brain lobes varied more than 3 MHz, a headache would begin. By comparison, if the frequency varied more than 10 MHz, a migraine headache would develop.

In creating an essential oil formula composed of Helichrysum, Chamomile and Lavender, to be inhaled by the recipient, Dr. Young discovered that the frequency of the head could be balanced, returning to normal within a few seconds.

Pure, unadulterated, essential oils start at 52 MHz and move upwards to as high as 320 MHz, which is the frequency of rose oil.

Clinical research continues to show that essential oils have the highest frequency of any natural substance for creating an environment in which disease, bacteria and viruses cannot exist. One can easily begin to make the connection that appears to exist between keeping the frequency of the body high enough (and well oxygenated) to be free of disease.

Science is just now re-discovering the incredible healing power of essential oils, the very lifeblood of the plant kingdom, the liquid that is extracted from flowers, trees, leaves, roots, shrubs, bushes and seeds. In summation, they are the "immune system" of the plant itself.

Clearly, this is an area in which much additional research is warranted.

By my very nature, I am a researcher. I am also an avid reader. It was in my travels that I chanced across a book by Luc Bourgault called *The American Indian Secrets of Crystal Healing*. The reading so impressed me that I am hereby sharing some insightful quotes.

To begin with, the first crystal with which you work, which you clean, polish and purify, must be yourself. It is an illusion to think that you can work effectively with crystals if you have not already started to work on yourself. [16]

You must understand that the crystal is a tool. It is not the crystal which will do the work but the person who holds it and who channels their will to heal into it. [17] **If you do not purify the crystal that is you, it is wrong to believe you will obtain beneficial results from crystal therapy.** [18]

---

[16] Bourgault, Luc. (1996). *The American Indian Secrets of Crystal Healing* (p 17). UK: W. Foulsham & Co. Ltd.
[17] Ibid, p 18.
[18] Ibid.

Meditation, prayer and physical exercises are all appropriate means of achieving purification of, and control over, one's thoughts, feelings, words and gestures. [19]

It is important to understand that we are all like a great lake, where all our thoughts are waves which reach many people before touching the shore and returning to us. Thus, if you have a bad thought about someone, it will touch that person and subsequently come back to you. You must therefore be very careful about what you think. [20]

Meditation and work on yourself, these must provide the basis of your efforts before you attempt to use crystals. Your spiritual path will take you everywhere in life. [21]

... crystals are living beings and an intimate part of the Earth. [22]

Everything that we think, say and do is registered, expressed and amplified by the crystals. If you possess a

---

[19] Bourgault, Luc. (1996). *The American Indian Secrets of Crystal Healing* (p 18). UK: W. Foulsham & Co. Ltd.
[20] Ibid, p 19.
[21] Ibid.
[22] Ibid, p 21.

power such as that of working with crystals, you have also the responsibility for it. With any power there comes responsibility. [23]

Crystals are the eyes, the ears, the nose and the mouth of the Earth, which uses them to see, to hear, to smell and to taste. It is also through them that it communicates with its other brothers and sisters, with other planets in the solar system. Each crystal taken from the Earth maintains its contact with the heart of the Earth. In many ways crystals are a little like *the eye of God*, communicating to the heavens and the Earth the thoughts and actions of humanity. [24]

... we must be very meticulous about the way in which we use crystals. [25]

It is very important to think about the health of Mother Earth when working with crystals, because one is manipulating some very private parts of her body. She is quite happy to accept this form of crystalline life, so one must respect it by respecting each crystal, which belongs

---

[23] Bourgault, Luc. (1996). *The American Indian Secrets of Crystal Healing* (p 24). UK: W. Foulsham & Co. Ltd.
[24] Ibid.
[25] Ibid.

to her body. **Significantly, the American Indians call stones and crystals** *the bones of Mother Earth.* [26]

Crystals are very powerful tools and it is possible to make mistakes if a) they are wrongly used, b) you are not in a state of perfect balance, or c) you are not able to sense correctly the level of healing which the person you are treating can cope with, both physically and spiritually. With your hands, however, it is impossible to make such mistakes. [27]

Your hands are natural healing instruments which are adaptable and allow the people you are treating to draw only what they need from you. It is therefore particularly beneficial to learn how to use your hands properly for healing before working with crystals. [28]

Indeed, Luc's words are most powerful, thereby meriting careful rereading and significant reflection.

In fact, before reading any further, I suggest that you take some time to thoroughly reflect on the words shared herein, *feeling what they mean to you.*

---

[26] Bourgault, Luc. (1996). *The American Indian Secrets of Crystal Healing* (pp 24-25). UK: W. Foulsham & Co. Ltd.
[27] Ibid, p 69.
[28] Ibid.

My Final Exam

What follows below is my final Crystal Healing Practitioner exam, in its entirety. I trust that it shall be of benefit to you, the reader.

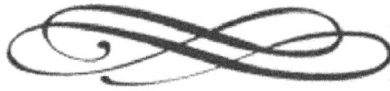

The therapeutic use of gems is not a new or alternative healing method.

Evidence that gemstones were used to heal disease can be found from the most ancient civilizations. Whether in leather pouches as carried by the Sumerians, or worn as talismans and amulets, or distilled into powders for elixirs, gemstones were known by natural healers to strengthen those who wore them, protecting them from evil spirits, sickness and disaster.

In the Vedic tradition, naturopathic medicine was known as Ayurveda, a word that is derived from sanskrit with ayur meaning life and veda meaning wisdom. This system of naturopathic medicine describes in detail how to prepare elixirs, pastes and powders made from gemstones.

In the first Chinese medical book, written 5000 years ago by Shen Nung, the Red Emperor, can be found detailed descriptions of gemstones and their influence on the body.

Quartz is a medium through which energies can be amplified. That having been said, it matters naught if the energy is positive or negative.

Crystals, when they come into your possession, can still be holding programs that allow them to work with discordant energies. Deprogramming stops the crystals from doing this.

There is a difference between programming and cleaning or cleansing.

Programming imprints a command, or a thought form or idea, into the internal matrix of the crystal, just as you would put the information onto the hard disk of a computer. Clearing and cleansing merely clears the crystal of the accumulation of unwanted energies.

Despite the fact that the most commonly given method of deprogramming and cleansing one's crystal is to put them in sea salt or saline solutions, I choose specifically not to use this method.

I choose not to avail of this method for the simple reason that salt is a crystalline structure. It is also a great gatherer of discordant energies, or energies that have disassociated themselves from the Source, or from the Light.

Crystals do not like salt because it gets into the microscopic cracks in the faces of the crystal and leeches out their water content. They dehydrate and start to crack. It is possible to actually deprogram and reprogram the salt in order to clear it of unwanted energies, but even so the crystals still do not like being in salt, because of the dehydration that it causes.

I clear and cleanse my crystals, before using, with intent. Thought is energy, and intent is everything. When you draw a symbol in your mind, or with your hands, or repeat the name of a symbol, then you link, or connect with, the energy of that symbol. This is linked with intent.

I therefore make use of my Reiki 2 symbols, first connecting by invoking the Choku Rei (three times) followed by the Sei Hei Ki, to clear of accumulated energies (three times). I then follow with the Choku Rei (three times), repeating twice more in succession.

Just as there are different categories associated with gemstones, so, too, are there different uses associated with each.

ROUGH stones (allowed to remain in their natural condition), understandably, are said to possess the greatest healing power and should be placed directly upon the body.

TUMBLED stones are more gentle and calming in nature; often used as touchstones, they are best suited for a number of purposes; namely, to be laid or pressed into the body; holding them; rubbing them; placing them directly under one's pillow; worn over clothing.

PRECIOUS and SEMI-PRECIOUS stones are most often crafted into jewelry. The metals in which these stones are set can increase their energy level.

There are many different methods of utilizing the powers of individual crystals, as indicated above, for healing purposes.

I enjoy placing crystals within my environment to (a) soak up electromagnetic pollution (related to computer, microwave, mobile phone, and television) and to (b) bring peace and harmony to an area.

Crystals have the property of trying to instill order into whatever place they are put, so handling or being surrounded by crystals will always have a beneficial effect.

In my attempt to oxygenate the air in a stagnant room, I will place numerous crystal clusters about the area.

I have begun meditating with stones resting on my body in the belief that my awareness will connect with the attributes of the stone, thereby inviting the crystal deva (spirit) into my life.

There exists a popular trend towards programming a crystal to fulfill a specific purpose. I am most uncomfortable with this practice, having wondered if such might actually have an adverse effect on the crystal, myself and anyone upon whom the stone might be used, for it is in programming a crystal that one attempts to exert their will on the deva.

Is this not akin to enslaving the free spirit (consciousness) of the crystal?

One merely has to stop for a moment to consider if they would wish to be treated in such a manner. To my way of thinking, there is no doubt that in acting contrary to the rule of harm none, there could be negative repercussions.

In addition to wearing crystal jewelry, I carry crystals and stones around with me (inside my deerskin medicine pouch), believing that I can draw upon their energies and attributes as needed. In making my selection, I focus on the key metaphysical properties attributed to each.

I enjoy meditating within a crystal field (placing crystals around my body) while seated on the floor.

I make use of my chakra disks (imported from the UK) to help clear my chakras. In a healthy body, each of these energy vortexes revolves at great speed, permitting vital life energy to flow upward. When energy is blocked in a specific chakra, symptoms develop in the associated organ or bodily system. The quickest way to regain youth, health and vitality is to assist these energy centers in spinning normally.

One of the simplest ways to help balance the whole chakra system is to place a stone of the appropriate colour on each area of the body. It is also a good idea to place a grounding stone between the feet to act as an anchor. One may also elect to visualize colour in the area of the chakra while holding specific stones and listening to chakra clearing meditations. As the chakras open, one gains better health, emotional balance and vitality.

In addition to the seven basic chakras, there are three major energy flow points that healers can avail of. They are (a) the Soul Star (located above the Crown chakra), (b) the Earth Star (located below the feet and within the Earth), and (c) the Kundalini, which connects the Root chakra to the base of the brain.

I have also come across additional interchangeable terms; namely, Transpersonal chakra for Soul Star and Earth chakra for Earth Star.

The function of the Soul Star is to connect our energies with the potent forces of the Universe. The function of the Earth Star is to connect our energies with Mother Earth in order to bring us to a greater understanding of the planet. The function of the Kundalini is to achieve fundamental cognitive change that can be utilized to drive the spiritual transformative process.

As there are specific colors associated with the seven basic chakras, so, too, are there organs associated with these energy flow points. Blockages cause disease which, then, causes most of our physical problems; hence, they must be removed. Crystals can help greatly in this regard.

It is important to realize that certain crystals also serve to balance the Yin and Yang energy meridians in the body. Malfunction, tension, disease and infection can result from an imbalance in the energy distribution along the meridian system. Given that vital energy (chi) flows via the meridian system from one organ to another, it must flow freely in order to maintain and promote optimum physical functioning and good health.

An imbalance in a specific meridian does not necessarily mean that there is something wrong with the organ associated with that meridian. Rather, it implies that there is either too much or too little energy along that meridian. One's first duty is to make the body healthy.

When conducting Reiki treatments, I strap slender Lemurian crystals to my wrists (placing them inside athletic bands) with the points facing downwards. Using one on each wrist, of about the same size, will amplify the universal healing energy (also known as pure, unconditional love) that flows during the session.

It is also my intention to further combine these two healing modalities in other intuitive ways.

There are a multitude of crystal layouts that I am able to avail of for balancing and calming, alleviating stress and tension, centering and grounding my energies, soothing headaches, easing PMT and menstrual cramps, relieving aches and pains and energizing my body.

As a means of energizing, cleaning and clearing one's aura and meridians, I often lie on my bed with clear crystal points facing inwards for about 10 minutes.

It is then followed up by reversing the crystals, so that their points are now facing outwards, thereby drawing off all unwanted energies, lowering high temperatures, drawing away any inflammation. I remain in this position for about 10 minutes.

The session is completed by turning the crystals inward, thereby re-energizing and balancing my body once more.

Many people say that dowsing is difficult, and that it requires certain gifts or skills in order to be a dowser, but it is actually the easiest thing in the world.

We are all human tuning forks, receiving and transmitting a myriad of energies and frequencies continuously, and the reply to your questions in dowsing will come through your I AM presence (also known as your Higher Self).

I make use of several pendulums. In asking questions, one must be as clear and precise as possible. Just formulate the thought in your mind, with intention, and allow the impressions to flow through you, holding the pendulum with an impartial mind. Ask the question, and then empty your mind, and take the answer that you get. If you think that you have not received an accurate answer, then you can always reconfirm it again by slightly re-wording your question.

One can ask questions about choosing crystals and identifying blocked chakras.

In summary, in order to fully appreciate the value of working with crystals in healing, it is important to recognize that the human body is basically crystalline in nature (water and blood are both forms of liquid crystal).

The blood, for example, with the help of intention, could be reprogrammed to become living crystal light, carried to every part and cell of the body, encoded with the energies of the blueprint of creation in accordance with Divine Will (utilizing only energies that are of the Light) for one's evolution in this lifetime.

Clearly, crystals can be seen as a means of aiding the healing of both our physical bodies as well as the consciousness of our cellular structure.

When you stop to consider the implications of this, it opens up a whole new avenue of possibilities.

Hand Brushing

There are chakras in the palms of your hands and the tips of your fingers. These can be activated to increase sensitivity. This is useful in the healing arts as well as in sensing the energies of your crystals.

First, lightly and quickly rub your hands together briskly, palm to palm. Continue this brushing motion for about 30 seconds.

To activate the fingertips, put the tips of your left fingers against the tips of your right fingers, rubbing them briskly but lightly together. Continue for about one minute. As there are many meridian, or energy, lines at the tips of your fingers, this may also create a sense of overall well-being.

Upon the completion of these exercises, you will have energized (and sensitized) your touching abilities.

Spread your hands about 6 inches apart, palms facing one another. You may now feel a pressure between your hands. Slowly move your hands slightly closer before pulling away again. What do you feel?

Try using a fingertip, moving it in a circular pattern a few inches away from the palm of the other hand. How does this feel?

If you are not getting any response, you may wish to begin this activity from the beginning again. With a little practice, you will begin to sense your hand energies. What you are engaged in feeling is the energy field from each hand brushing up against the other.

Choosing Your Crystals

To select a crystal, put yourself in a calm, relaxed and centered space. Hold the crystal in your left hand (the receiving hand), feeling it physically and emotionally. Feel the energy from the stone.

Close your eyes, breathe deeply and regularly. Be open to any sensations like tingling, goose bumps, even a change in temperature. If you feel that nothing is happening, quickly do a Hand Brushing exercise to activate your palm chakras.

Feel and see if you feel attracted to it. Allow the crystal to pick you!

Some people choose stones based on the metaphysical properties associated with them, as may be the basis of many a personal experience when not in areas where one can actually physically handle a crystal.

Different color stones offer strengths and areas upon which you can focus. The darker the stone, the denser and more earthy (grounding) the stone.

If it is in one's nature to day dream, with thoughts flying about, one may need the stabilizing effects of the physically grounding stones.

If one is naturally grounded, stable and methodical lighter stones (clear quartz, white or violet stones) will stimulate imagination, clarity and inspiration.

If one is still unsure as to which to choose, one can always relate crystals to the colors within the chakras. In this light, it is valuable to develop an understanding of the key seven energy centers (chakras). This knowledge can be used to assist one in many areas of their life.

Always *remember to go with your initial gut feeling* when making your choice.

Cleansing of Crystals

Despite the fact that the most commonly given method of cleansing crystals is to put them in salt, sea salt or saline solutions, I *do not* recommend this. Please refer back to the segment called My Final Exam (on page 15) for reasons specific to crystals.

How, then, do we clear and cleanse our crystals? We do it with intent, as discussed within this segment. It is important to realize that *thought is energy*, and *intent is everything.*

Here are a few additional ways to cleanse your crystals

[1] Energizing your crystal in the moonlight is very popular. Leaving your crystal out for a 24 hour period under a full moon is even better.

[2] Run it under purified water. If there are points on your stone, make sure that they point downward to let the negativity run down the drain. However, this would not be appropriate for all stones, as some will dissolve in water.

[3] You can bury your stones in the ground (clearly marked area) for a 24 hour period. Apartment dwellers can reap similar benefits from burying the stones in organic potting soil for the same amount of time. Do not use for iron based stones such as Hematite and Tiger Eye.

[4] There are Tibetan Prayer Bowls made of metal alloy (looks like brass) that resonate when struck or rubbed along the rim. These bowls can hold many stones at once. They are cleansed thoroughly and quickly (within a minute or so). The sound also has a purifying effect on the surroundings.

[5] Smudging is the least invasive and most popular method for clearing gemstones. You can use a smudge stick for this. A smudge stick may consist of some of the following herbs: cedar, sage, lavender, juniper or pine. You can either pass your gemstones through the smoke or pass the smudge stick over them. This method is excellent for clearing yourself and your environment as well.

[6] Placing your stones on a Quartz cluster while also positioning four single terminated Quartz points around the cluster is an easy method. Creating a cross formation around the cluster, place the single crystals in north, south, east and west directions. In this way the single points charge the cluster which, in turn, recharges the stones.

It is very reassuring to note that Quartz clusters themselves rarely need cleansing due to the intense light reflection off of the terminated points, which, in turn, creates a force field that is self-energizing.

[7] Charging your stones inside the base of a stand-upright copper energizing pyramid that has been built with the sacred geometry ratios of the Great Pyramids at Giza is an excellent method to avail of.

[8] For those who are at least Level 2 Reiki practitioners, you can also invoke several Reiki symbols. Holding the crystal in my left hand, I begin by reciting the Choku Rei (three times), followed by the Sei He Ki (three times), and lastly, once again, by the Choku Rei (three times). I then repeat the entire process twice.

We must continue to realize that we are healing facilitators and not healers.

When conducting Reiki client treatments, I strap crystals to my wrists (placing them inside athletic bands) with the points facing downwards. Using one on each wrist, of about the same size, will amplify the universal healing energy (also known as pure, unconditional love) that flows during the session.

When conducting long-distance Reiki sessions, as before, I strap crystals to my wrists (placing them inside athletic bands), this time positioning the points facing upwards as my hands are positioned in a position of giving thanks. As before, using one on each wrist, of about the same size, will amplify the universal healing energy that flows during the session.

It is always the recipient who is the healer, working directly with the universal energies directed their way, all in an effort to heal themselves.

Crystals are capable of holding very precise and steady frequencies. This is why crystals are used in mobile telephones, radio transmitters and receivers, quartz watches, etc.

Crystals have within them spiral matrixes, some spiraling to the left and some to the right. We therefore refer to the crystal as right or left-handed, or a male or female crystal, although many prefer not to use gender terms. You will need to look for the direction in which the smallest face of the crystal is formed.

If the face is pointing straight up, this indicates that the crystal can be used in either hand, and is a neutral channeler of energy.

If the face is leaning to the right, or left, then it follows that this is either a right handed or left handed crystal. Some of them have various angles to these slanting faces. The sharper the angle, the more orientated towards the right or left hand it becomes.

Sometimes, you will find a crystal that has both a small face that leans to the right, as well another that leans to the left. In this case the crystal has a double spiral, and can be used in either hand.

Left handed crystals, used in your left hand, will take away energy and inflammation; whilst right handed crystals, used in your right hand, will increase energy. Where the spiral is pointing straight up, then the crystal is very balanced, and can be used for either of these purposes. We can use crystals as energizing tools in our hands.

After choosing your crystal, you may want to spend some time exploring it.

Crystals can be used to heal an individual on all levels (spiritual, mental, emotional and physical). This is possible because of the body's frequencies of energy waves. Crystals naturally work with this energy. The crystal taps into the body's energy waves (including chakras) and proceeds to correct and transmit the healing frequency back to the human energy field.

Crystals can clear stagnant energy from a room by absorbing positive ions.

Placed on, or near, appliances such as computers, televisions and microwaves, a crystal can absorb potentially harmful rays.

House plants will benefit from a crystal placed in the top of their pots. Jade is said to amplify the energies of the plant while Turquoise will help the plant recover from damage and disease.

The ability to be effective in learning situations depends upon several factors that can be enhanced by the use of crystals.

The mind needs to be clear, focused and alert. Clear Quartz brings stillness to the mind, and a grounding stone prevents your mind from straying. Take the Quartz into a test or examination. It will remind you of what you have learned and will give you extra confidence and clarity.

The colour yellow is known to stimulate the logical functions of the mind, so a bright yellow stone like Amber, Citrine or Fluorite will assist memory and recall. Any sort of Fluorite is an excellent stone for study as it helps to balance the functioning of the brain hemispheres. This is particularly helpful when you need to do a lot of reading.

Deep blue stones, like Kyanite, Sodalite and Sapphire, will enable clearer communication skills and better understanding of ideas and concepts.

Pyramids create large powerful energy fields around them and are useful for energizing a healing room or other large spaces.

Crystals are often worn for protection or enhancement of a particular area in one's life.

You can carry them about in your pocket. They can be kept on a desk in front of you at your place of work. They can also be put under your pillow at night.

Taking the time to explore crystals is useful in developing your sensitivity to their subtle energy fields. Having cleansed your crystal, you are ready to begin. Please be sure to denote any sensations that you may experience while attempting crystal energy exploration techniques.

Do you feel coolness? Do you feel heat?

Does it pulse gently? Are your fingertips tingling?

Do you feel invigorated or soothed by its presence in your hand or on your body?

Has your heart started to beat more quickly?

Have your shoulders dropped and your neck muscles softened as you hold the stone?

Do you feel comfortable holding it or are you feeling slightly off balance?

It is important that you *keep questioning* how you feel.

The Wisdom of Crystals

FIRST EXPERIENCES

The crystals I were initially drawn to (color, size, shape)

_____

_____

_____

_____

_____

_____

_____

_____

_____

FIRST EXPERIENCES

My first crystal and why I chose it

_____

_____

_____

_____

_____

_____

_____

_____

_____

_____

_____

FIRST EXPERIENCES

My first experience of tuning into my crystal involved

_____

_____

_____

_____

_____

_____

_____

_____

_____

_____

_____

LATER EXPERIENCES

The crystals I choose to have around me (list them)

_____

_____

_____

_____

_____

_____

_____

_____

_____

_____

_____

LATER EXPERIENCES

Different ways I have experimented with my crystals

_____

_____

_____

_____

_____

_____

_____

_____

_____

_____

_____

LATER EXPERIENCES

What worked well

_____

_____

_____

_____

_____

_____

_____

_____

_____

_____

_____

LATER EXPERIENCES

What did not work well

_____

_____

_____

_____

_____

_____

_____

_____

_____

_____

_____

LATER EXPERIENCES

How I felt when using crystals on my chakras

_____

_____

_____

_____

_____

_____

_____

_____

_____

_____

_____

[1] Look closely at your crystal. Feel the weight, shape and texture of the crystal. Close your eyes, holding it in both hands for a minute or two.

[2] Hold the crystal in both hands close to the solar plexus. As you exhale, imagine your breathe passing over the top of the stone. As you inhale, see your breathe entering the crystal and being drawn into your body. The breath creates a cycle passing from you through the crystal and back into your body. Continue this breathing cycle to build up energy, then relax. This is an easy and effective way to integrate a crystal's energy into your own energy.

[3] Place the crystal on a surface a comfortable distance in front of you. Sit quietly with your eyes closed for a moment. Open your eyes. Look at the crystal before you. Close your eyes and sit quietly for a minute or two. Reach out and pick up the crystal. Hold it in both hands for a little while with your eyes closed. After a minute or two, place the stone back in front of you. Repeat this picking up and putting down several times and make note of any changes in how you feel.

[4] Hold your stone in your left hand for several moments. Put the stone down and pick up with your right hand. Repeat this process several times. Do you notice any changes in what you feel as you go from hand to hand?

[5] Lie down and place the stone on different chakra centers. Usually the solar plexus, heart and brow (third eye) are the most sensitive.

[6] Take three clear quartz crystals with naturally terminated points and try each of the following in sequence, spending two or three minutes on each.

Place all three crystals, evenly spaced, next to the left side of the body. Start with all the crystals pointed in toward you, and after a minute or two, turn their points away from your body.

Put all three crystals next to the right side of your body. Start with all the crystals pointed in toward you, and after a minute or two, turn their points away from your body.

Try all three stones placed around your head. Start with all the crystals pointed in toward you, and after a minute or two, turn their points away from your body.

Follow this by positioning the quartz crystals, points down, below your feet.

You will probably notice a difference in sensations within the body. Perhaps your mind will become quieter or busier than usual, your breathing may alter.

Make a note of your experiences, even if it is as vague as feeling comfortable or fidgety. When you have clear results, try with the same stones, but this time place them on your body and see how your experiences differ.

Crystal Visualization Exercises

[1] Sit (or lie down) in a comfortable position, holding your stone. Take time to relax. Focus on feeling the cosmic energy above and all around you. Focus on feeling the cosmic energy flowing through you. Feel your body as the cosmic energy sweeps up and down your arms and into the hands that are holding the crystal.

[2] Slowly let your awareness float down into the crystal until you reach a point where you seem to come to a rest. Now you should feel the energy as it flows through the crystal (and out through the tip, which should be pointed away from you).

[3] Notice what you feel as the energy surges through from your hand to your crystal. Does your hand suddenly feel hotter or colder?

[4] If your crystal has a point you may try this. Very gently place the crystal so that the tip points toward the back of your hand. Position the crystal so that it remains about 2 feet away. As it hits the back of your hand, are you able to feel the energy in a fine focused line?

49

If you cannot feel anything, slowly bring the crystal toward your hand. When is it that you start to feel something?

[5] Concentrate on the flow of cosmic energy through you and into the crystal. Can you feel a sudden energy surge? Put the crystal on your lap and send energy from one hand to the other in the same position as before. Is there a sudden drop in energy flow? Pick up the crystal and compare.

[6] When you have finished, remember to cleanse both yourself and the stone. Focus on the weight of your body or feet if they are on the floor. Feel yourself get heavier while still remaining aware of the world around you. Take some notes so that you can remember your experiences.

Color is an indicator of one of the characteristics of energy. Color is a primary identification factor that links crystals and gemstones to their best uses.

The visible light spectrum goes from the lowest frequency (red) to the highest (violet). This spectrum, in order: red, orange, green, blue, indigo and violet.

Colors also correspond with our body's energy centers (chakras) by way of frequency (low to high). The lowest frequency center in the body is the Root or Base chakra, which is influenced greatly by the color red, the lowest color frequency.

Color rays affect our physical bodies, our emotions and our moods.

RED

Red is the primary color of the Root chakra, or energy center located at the base of the spine, that connects us to the Earth and our physical reality. Our physical relationship with the color red connects at the legs, feet, hips and base of the spine. On a mental level, red energy manifests itself as assertiveness and self-confidence and, when out of balance, aggression and arrogance.

Red energy is always needed at the beginning of any creative venture. Being grounded, focused, realistic and in contact with the Earth, as well as the physical body, shows a balance of red within an individual. The best way to balance red energy is to allow it to flow.

There are many red stones, including Garnet, Ruby, Spinel, Zircon, Jasper, Red Quartz, Red Tourmaline, Hematite and Granite.

The ability to succeed, demonstrating skill in the manipulation of physical things, being down-to-earth and business like are all manifestations of red energy.

Indicators of a <u>lack</u> or red energy include	An <u>excess</u> of red energy might manifest as
• cold, inactive, congested conditions	• hyperactivity
• difficulty with physical movement	• inflammation
• circulation problems	• physical tension
• inability to sustain energy levels	• inability to relax
• physical weakness and exhaustion	• anger
• lacking in drive and enthusiasm	• fear
• lethargic	• emotional/mental confusion
• feelings of vulnerability and alienation	• rapid mood swings
	• impatience
	• fidgeting
	• intolerance
	• violent outbursts

ORANGE

Orange is the energy of red modified by yellow. Any injury, shock or trauma, whether life-threatening or transitory, whether physical, emotional or mental, whether in the distant past or the present, can be dissolved and healed with the help of orange.

Orange vibration stimulates and encourages creativity on all levels, for the same reason that it is effective in healing, because it helps to remove any blockage in the way of growth.

Orange energy is related to the energy and functions of the second Sacral chakra situated within the pelvic area. The organs within the lower abdomen, especially the large intestine and the reproductive organs, as well as the kidneys higher in the abdominal cavity, all carry out orange type activities. Orange at the emotional level works positively with creativity and negatively with stress.

Orange stones include Tiger Eye, Dark Citrine Quartz, Copper, Sunstone, Golden Topaz, Orange Calcite, Carnelian and Amber.

A <u>lack</u> of orange energy might manifest as	The nature of the orange vibration means that it is unusual to find a build up of excess energy.
• physical rigidity	
• restricted feelings	
• digestive disorders	
• lack of focus	
• lack of vitality	
• being stuck in the past (holding onto memories)	

YELLOW

Yellow is the color of the sun, and, like the sun, yellow energy tends to make us feel happy and in harmony with our surroundings. At a physical level, the yellow vibration is associated with the Solar Plexus chakra and with the upper abdomen. Many other physical systems, such as the immune system, rely on the yellow vibration. The yellow energy expresses intelligence and clarity.

Emotionally, yellow energy positively translates as feelings of joy, happiness and contentment. Negatively, it becomes fear, worry, anxiety and panic. The source of these negative emotions is usually confusion and lack of knowledge. We panic because we lack the right information to know what to do next. Once there is a clear idea of what we can do, confusion vanishes and choices become clear. Yellow emotional states are thus a response to our mental state. Where yellow energy is strong, there is clear knowledge of who one is and how to interact with the world.

Iron Pyrite (also called Fool's Gold), Gold, Amber, Light Citrine Quartz, Lemon Quartz, Yellow Sapphire, Yellow Jasper, Helidor (Yellow Beryl) and Yellow Fluorite are some of the more common yellow stones.

Physical imbalances of yellow energy might manifest as	An excess of yellow mental energy could be exhibited as
• stress related ailments (indigestion, insomnia, panic attacks, headaches, muscle tension)	• overanalytical, fussy behavior
• skin complaints (eczema, psoriasis)	• narrow conceptual categorizations
• nervous disorders	• prejudices
• allergic reactions	• lack of tolerance
• food intolerance	
• arthritis	
• tension	
• worry	
• confusion	

GREEN

Green is found in the middle of the color spectrum. Green is the primary color of vegetation and has associations with life, growth and the world of nature. Green is the color of harmonious balance, a calming, restful energy that is linked with the central chakra, the Heart. Physically, green is associated with the heart, lungs, diaphragm and the arms and hands. The functions of respiration, growth and the ability to change and adapt are closely linked with this color.

Green is associated with our personal space and a sense of freedom with the ability, or lack of ability, to express ourselves from the heart. The basis of green energy is the need to grow, expand and increase our influence and power.

At a physical level, green links all of the systems and organs of the body that maintain balance. At an emotional level, green reflects the balance within the heart. Loving, caring and sharing are the expansive, inclusive qualities of this color, expanding the self by establishing relationships with others. Mentally, green energy gives structure to our existence. Spiritually, the green vibration relates to all aspects of personal growth and the ability to discern and travel our own personal road.

Green Aventurine, Jade, Peridot, Malachite, Green Tourmaline, Green Calcite, Moss Agate, Emerald and Dioptase are all examples of green stones.

Green <u>imbalances</u> include anything that intrudes into or restricts personal boundaries and equilibrium

• invasive illness

• abnormal growths

• lack of control at any level

• sense of claustrophobia

• feeling unfulfilled/restricted/dominated

• a need to be in control or to be controlled

• lack of self-discipline

• confusion as to who one is and what direction should be taken

• feelings of isolation

BLUE AND INDIGO

Blue is about flow and communication on all levels. Whenever there is a build-up of tension, a sensation of friction or frustration, a blockage of energies, blue light will restore the flow. Blue is the antidote to any over concentration of energy, making it the opposite to red light in this respect.

Physically, the color blue connects with the Throat and Brow (third eye) chakras. It covers the neck, throat, face, ears, eyes, nose, mouth and forehead. All forms of communication, expression and learning are blue in quality. At an emotional level, the color blue can create a flow that helps understanding, empathy, appreciation and acceptance. It is a color that can reduce the irritation we feel when something jars against our own preferences or beliefs. By increasing our ability to communicate with others and express ourselves effectively, the blue energy can prevent the build up of friction that would otherwise develop into a red condition of anger.

Self-expression and communication are basic human requirements. When there is an excess of blue energy, its coolness can become all-enveloping. Emotional detachment and aloofness are the result.

Blue is not a color to use in cases of depression, nor should it be used for extended periods without the balancing effect of more activating colors. Blue is a color that can increase our ability to contact the deep areas of the mind where inspiration and imagination reside. It allows intuition to flourish.

Some examples of *Light Blue* stones are Celestite, Blue Topaz, Blue Lace Agate, Angelite, Aquamarine and Blue Calcite. These are the stones that are more commonly linked to the Throat chakra.

Some examples of *Dark Blue*, or *Indigo*, stones are Lapis Lazuli, Sodalite, Blue Quartz, Blue Tourmaline, Kyanite, Sapphire and Azurite. These are the stones that are more commonly linked to the Brow (third eye) chakra.

Indicators of blue <u>imbalances</u> are

• throat problems (laryngitis, sore throats, tonsillitis)

• blocks to creativity and inspiration

• cold, congested states

Extreme agitated states can be helped with blue initially, although the calming qualities of green are more suitable in the long term.

VIOLET

The energy of violet is the synthesis of the hot, activating, dynamic manifesting quality of red with the cooling, sedating, pacifying, dematerializing color of blue.

The violet vibration relates to the Crown chakra and the head generally, but specifically the cranium or the skull. It also connects the functions of the brain to the pituitary and pineal glands within the physical body. Violet energy works to create coordination and integration between the physical systems. Physical condition problems and learning difficulties in children arise from an imbalance between the left and right hemispheres of the brain.

Violet is one of the most useful healing energies in crystal work. Violet energy at an emotional level tends to foster understanding and sympathy for others, and at a mental level opens the awareness to imagination and inspiration.

Violet encourages all aspects of artistic expression and practical problem solving. The expansive nature of the vibration also helps to enter and maintain meditative states.

Violet and/or purple stones include Amethyst Quartz, Purple Fluorite, Sugilite, Charoite, Iolite, Lepidolite and Violet Kunzite.

Violet energy imbalances can become extreme, expressing as	The following can be helped by violet energy
• exaggerated need to sacrifice for others (often disguises guilt and poor self-worth) • tendency to live in a world of illusion • delusional states	• headaches • problems with eyes and ears • deep seated glandular imbalances • chronic imbalances of the whole system • lack of mental focus • lack of spiritual focus • inability to concentrate

PINK

Pink is a combination of white and red and tends to be dynamic, expressing the energy and activation of red with the all-encompassing, cleansing qualities of white.

Jealousies, aggression and misunderstandings all fade away when illuminated by the pink vibration. Whenever there is a violent or negative situation, the use of pink light for short periods of time quickly reestablishes calm.

All issues to do with self-image can be greatly helped by the pink light.

Pink energy increases levels of tolerance and sympathy. It works well as first-aid and in the release of long-term trauma.

Rose Quartz, Pink Tourmaline (Rubellite), Rhodonite, Rhodochrosite, Pink Kunzite and Cherry Opal are all examples of pink stones.

TURQUOISE

Turquoise comes in a variety of shades between green and blue. The Heart center, represented by green energy, is linked together with the Throat chakra, the light blue energy, indicating that turquoise helps to articulate and express the true wishes of the heart.

Turquoise reaffirms our sense of value and purpose and significantly increases the life energy available to each of us. Consider using turquoise in any situation where stress and illness are clearly draining the individual.

Turquoise, Chrysocolla, Larimar, Gem Silica and Amazonite are examples of turquoise stones.

WHITE

White is the union of all colors, so it symbolizes the potential to reflect all energies. White is the vibration of pure potential. When combined with another color, white will amplify and augment that color.

White has no clear connection to the physical body, although it is often associated with the area just above the top of the head, at/or above the Crown chakra. Since it cannot absorb anything, it remains somewhat remote and inviolable; hence, its ties to purity.

It can be utterly cleansing, stripping away all masks and pretensions, so it should always be used with care.

Clear stones include Clear Quartz, Herkimer Diamond, Diamond, Iceland Spa, Gypsum, Selenite and Apophyllite.

Milky stones include Milky Quartz, Moonstone and Opal.

BLACK

Whereas white stones reflect and clarify light, black stones absorb all energies into itself so that no light can be seen. It contains within itself all potential, but where white will create energy for a rapid, immediate change of state, black will allow a rest period, a dormancy within which growth and change can begin to take shape.

Black can be a good grounding color, as their energy anchors to help you return to a normal state. Black can also be the means by which the underlying, hidden factors and emotions can be brought to the surface and examined.

Black is also a very protective color because it absorbs all energy, no matter what the source. In meditation, the color black can be extremely useful, creating a restful and tranquil silence in which it is possible to explore deep levels.

The combination of black and white can produce an extremely powerful blending of both protection and cleansing qualities.

Black Tourmaline (Schorl), Smoky Quartz, Obsidian, Jet and Onyx are examples of black stones.

Pendulum Dowsing

Pendulums have been used for thousands of years, becoming increasingly popular in Western society.

A Pendulum is any balanced weight suspended by a chain or thread, and is simply a means of visibly checking what the subconscious mind already knows.

The pendulum represents an extension of the inner senses and creates a visual representation of inner energy changes. The pendulum amplifies small muscle movements that result from changes in subtle energy flow through the physical body. The conscious mind, emotions and physical tension can all affect the pendulum.

Choose a pendulum with which you feel comfortable (well-balanced).

Keep the string about 4 to 5 inches long. Begin by holding the pendulum by the top of the string (cord or chain) between your thumb and index finger. Feel free to use either hand.

Take a couple of deep breaths, trying to have your arm, hands and fingers reasonably relaxed.

Without thinking too hard about it, ask your pendulum to swing in any direction for you. Do not consciously move your arm or hand as you do this. Using your thoughts alone will make the movement happen.

It does not matter if your pendulum begins to swing wildly, or it if just trembles slightly before going still. All you want is slight movement. Give yourself a good five minutes for this.

Whatever you accomplish in the early stages, know that you are not experiencing a mystical phenomenon, no matter how much it may feel that way. Unless the pendulum is in your hands, it will not move. It needs your energy interaction to move. Remember, your thought field generates in an area around you.

Many people say that dowsing is difficult, and that it requires certain gifts or skills in order to be a dowser, but it is actually the easiest thing in the world.

We are all human tuning forks, receiving and transmitting a myriad of energies and frequencies continuously, and the reply to your questions in dowsing will come through your I AM presence (also known as your Higher Self).

If you are interested in trying this method, then find yourself a pendulum.

This can be made either of a metal such as silver, gold, copper or pewter, or quartz crystal or mineral. Check by asking which way this particular pendulum moves to respond with a yes, and which way for a no.

You can then start asking your questions, as clearly and precisely as possible.

Just formulate the thought in your mind, again with intention, and allow the impressions to flow through you, holding the pendulum with an impartial mind. Ask the question, and then empty your mind, and take the answer that you get.

If you think that you have not received the accurate answer, then you can always reconfirm, or cross-confirm it, by slightly re-wording your question. You can also use this method of dowsing to check different crystal types, and what they are most suitable for.

Getting To Know Your Pendulum

With the crystal pendulum, you need to discover what each specific swing means to you. This will be unique to you.

Holding your pendulum in one hand, position your other palm facing upward; next, position your pendulum about 2 inches above your palm. Try to have your arm and hand nicely relaxed. Hold your elbow slightly away from your body, as if there were a tennis ball positioned in your armpit area.

When you are ready, ask your pendulum to show you YES. This will be a personal experience between you and your pendulum. It may remain motionless, it may swing back and forth, it may swing in a circle. Whatever happens, note its movement.

Repeat this same procedure, this time asking your pendulum to show you NO. This movement should be different. If it remains the same, firmly say "No" and once again request a different movement. Take your time and remember to keep breathing deeply.

When you are satisfied, go on to ask it to move in a direction that is NEUTRAL.

When you have completed this, you should have three distinct and firm movements.

Now you are ready to test your pendulum's truthfulness. Ask it a simple question to which the only answer can possibly be YES.

Note its response. Is it the right one? Keep questions simple and direct.

Mental and emotional neutrality can be easier to maintain if dowsing is done with lists, arcs, or with your free hands touching or pointing to stones.

Lists can be made of anything deemed useful to the healing facilitator.

Dowsing arcs are used instead of circles because any pendulum swing on a circle will pick out two sections at the top and bottom of the swing, but only one possible section is indicated on an arc.

Now that you have determined YES, NO and NEUTRAL, think of situations whereby you can use this information.

[1] You can use the pendulum to help guide you on practical matters such as allergies or reactions to certain foods. Do particular foods agree or disagree with you? Try placing your pendulum over particular foods and see what it tells you. You can also just write the name of the food on a piece of paper.

[2] You may want to decide which crystal, or which healing remedy, might work best for you. Try placing it over a variety of crystals and see which would be best for you.

[3] You can use it to make your own essential oil blends. Try asking it which oils would be good in a blend for you, and, of course, how many drops of each.

[4] You can find your color preferences for certain desires. Is this the best color for relaxation (creativity, stimulation, clarification, depression)? Do this by drawing a circle on a sheet of paper. Divide it into eight equal parts. Color the segments clockwise with the following colors: red, orange, yellow, green, turquoise, blue, indigo, violet.

[5] You can go through your chakras, one by one, asking your pendulum "Is my Root chakra being affected by this situation?"

These are but a few possibilities. Most of all, be creative.

PENDULUM WORK

My NEUTRAL means ......

_____

_____

_____

My YES means ......

_____

_____

_____

My NO means ......

_____

_____

_____

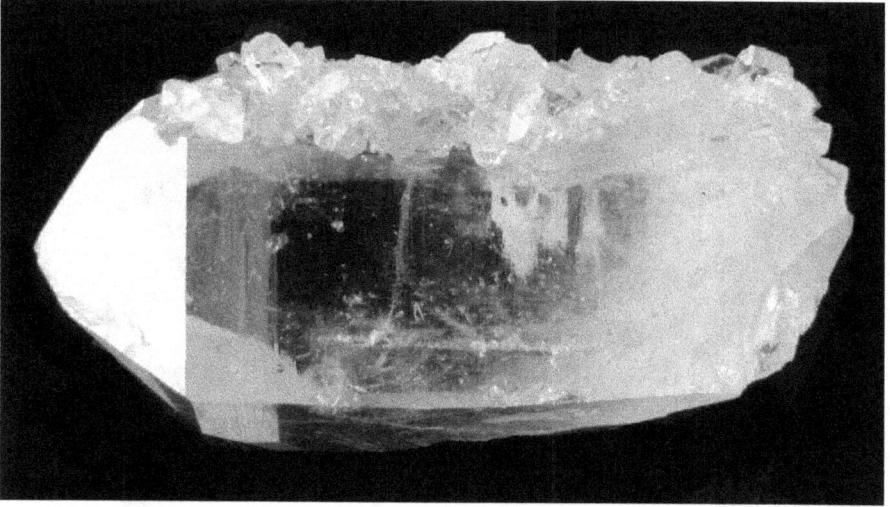

Barnacle Crystal – A large crystal covered, or partially covered, with smaller crystals. It is said that Barnacle crystals are helpful with family or group issues by providing cohesive group energy that enhances common purpose and thereby promotes the ability to work together.

Each time I spend time with a Barnacle crystal, I cannot help but compare its formation to that of a teacher (master) with many students wherein a combination of both teaching and learning is transpiring (in that each individual is both teacher and student).

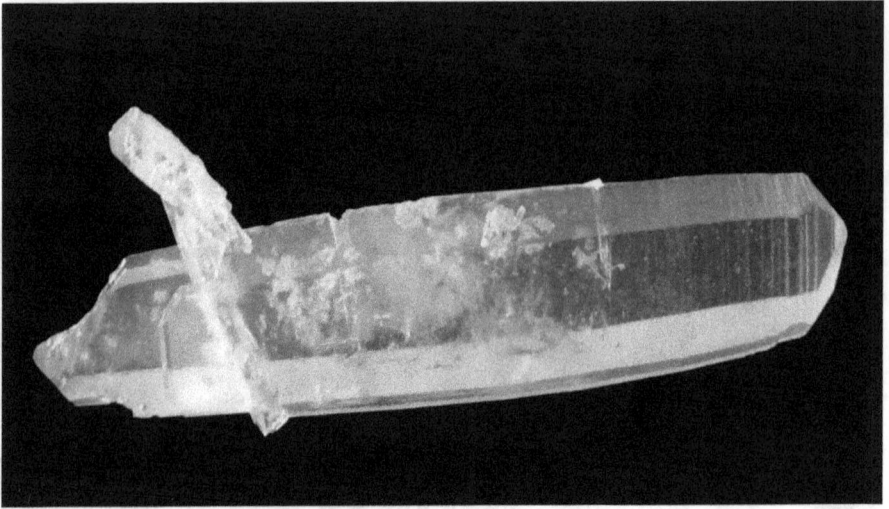

Bridge Crystal – Recognized by a smaller crystal(s) that either penetrates and/or is lodged partially, while still protruding outward from the main crystal. These crystals are considered, in a spiritual sense, to be the bridge between inner and outer worlds. Such is also transferrable to being the bridge between one's self and others.

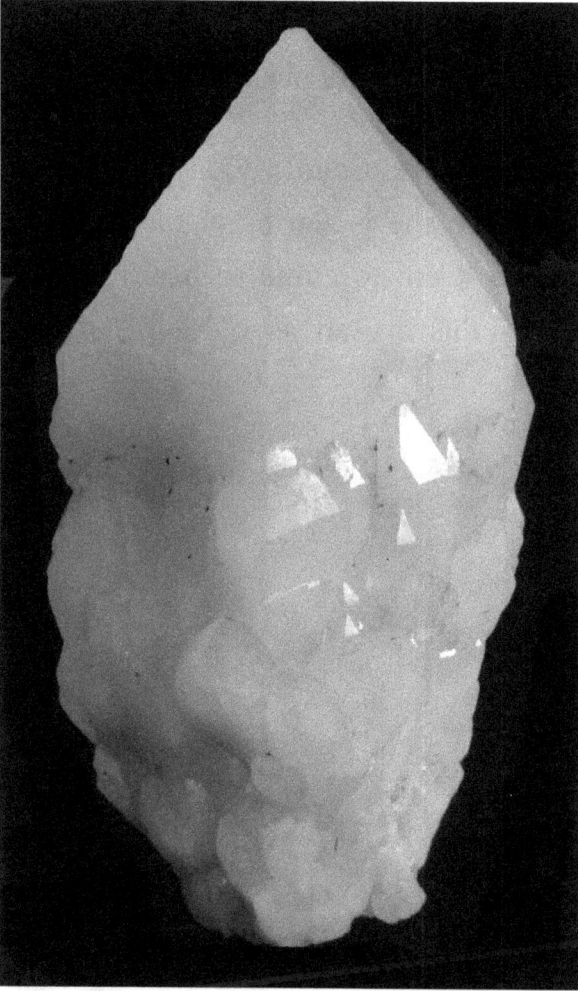

Candle Crystal – These crystals have a bumpy appearance (from hundreds of tiny crystals that coat the sides of the larger crystal) that reminds me of melted or dripping wax from a candle; hence, the name. This crystal has also been called Pineapple Quartz as well as Celestial Quartz.

Beautifully formed Candle Quartz allows us to look within and discover out true nature, our true path and true spirit.

Kellie Jo likes to use Candle Quartz for crystal gazing, meaning that while she is staring at the crystal, going over each facet, ideas seem to come to her, in endless fashion; hence, she uses this crystal as a means of enhancing her creativity.

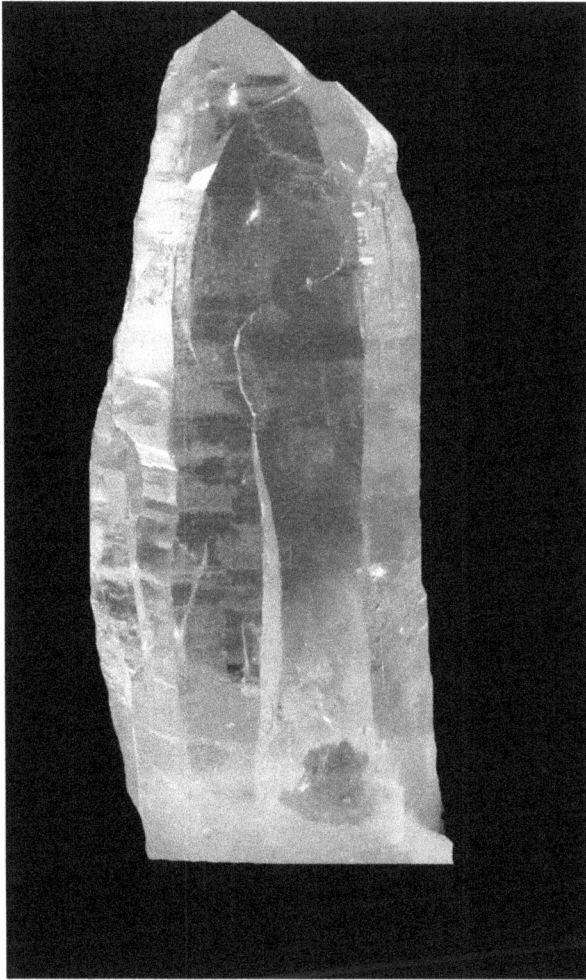

Cathedral Crystal – While these crystal pieces may appear to be composed of several separate pieces (which serve to create that parallel stepped or layered effect, whereby the formation is said to resemble cathedral organ pipes or spires), all are part of the main crystal (which has multiple terminations with at least one point at the apex).

Cathedral Quartz, the same as Cathedral Lightbrary Quartz, is touted as being the light worker and wisdom bearer extraordinaire of the crystal kingdom, more than likely because Cathedral Quartz is akin to a cosmic computer that contains the wisdom of the ages.

It is believed that Cathedral Quartz makes itself known every two thousand years to aid in the evolution of consciousness by raising thought to a higher vibration.

I have also come across the term Atlantis Temple Quartz as being the same as that of Cathedral Quartz; likewise for the term Castellated Quartz.

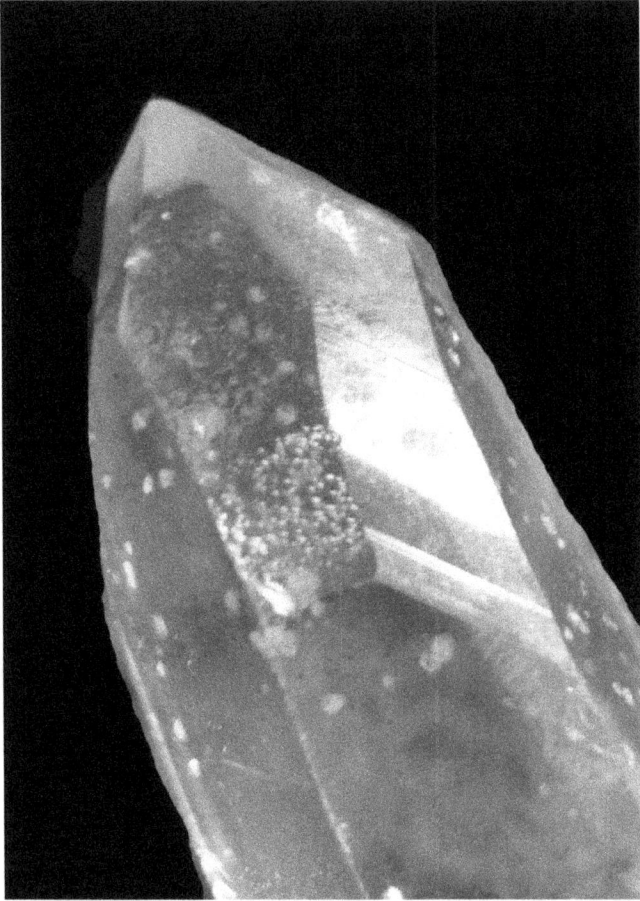

Chandelier Crystal – This is a new configuration coming out of Brazil. The most unusual feature of this crystal formation are the tiny diamond shaped facets around the termination (tip) of the crystal. These tiny facets resemble crystal shapes often seen dangling from a ceiling chandelier; hence, the name. In addition, there are multiple indentations, or tiny groups of indentations, which are more pronounced on certain crystal faces.

Chandelier crystals, as alluded to by their name, are bringers of light. As a result, they tend to enhance the light of their crystal guardian.

These crystals are now showing up, courtesy of both the new millennium as well as the fact that we are finally ready to explore our inner selves, discovering the divine spirit that lives within each soul. As a result, this crystal will enhance one's journey back to the knowingness that we are all spirit, that we are all connected, that we are all one.

We get there by surrendering to the one Source, to the *All That Is*, to God/dess, to the Higher Power, as guided by this single truth. It becomes in surrendering that we receive what is needed.

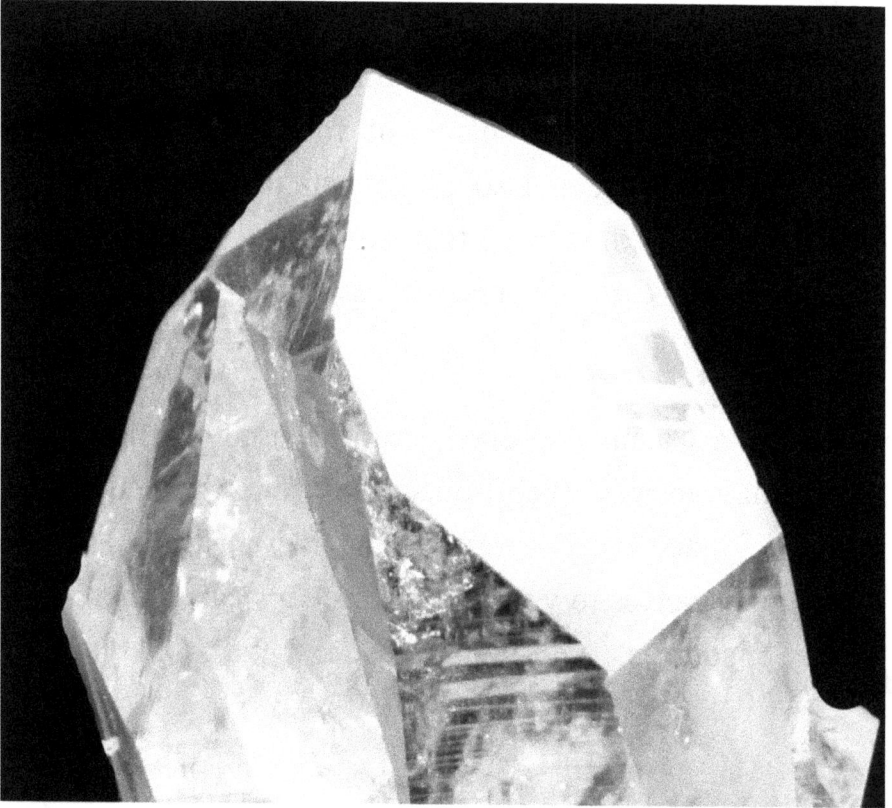

Channeling Crystal – These are recognized by their one large face, the other five faces being much smaller. The large face has seven sides. Its opposite, rear face, is a smaller triangle.

The number seven is said to represent wisdom and mysticism. It could be said that the triangle equates to our conscious mind, while the seven sided face is representative of the inner wisdom of the subconscious mind.

Channeling crystals are incredibly useful for obtaining information from deep within yourself, as well as from sources that are clearly outside of your normal 3D realm. As a result, they can also assist you in drawing on the information and knowledge that is provided by the universe (whereby you can also receive assistance from a higher source).

Likewise, a Channeling crystal can be used whenever you are seeking answers (help) outside of yourself. You must, however, listen very carefully for the answers as they present themselves to you because answers can come from a variety of sources.

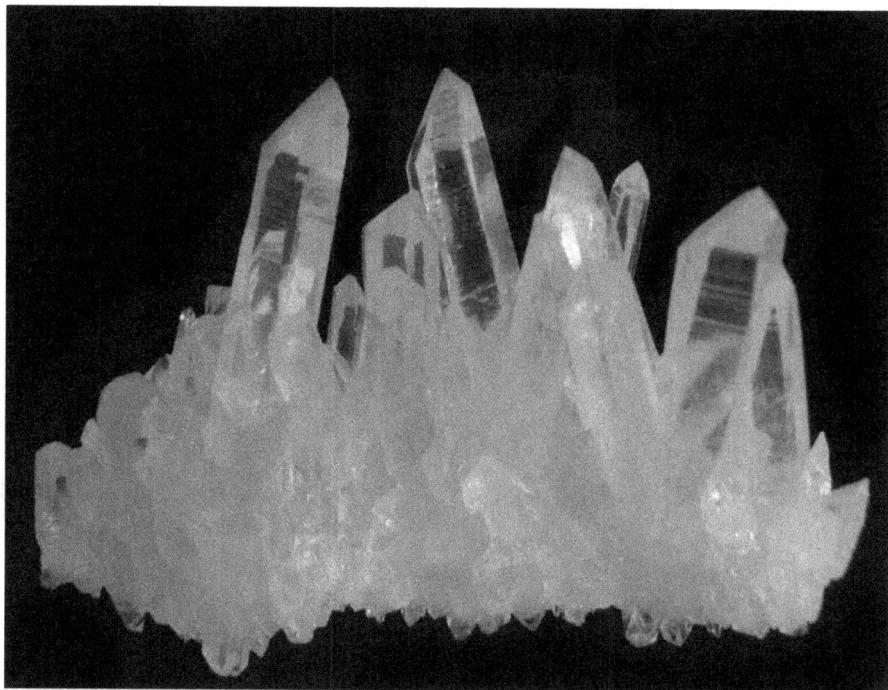

Crystal Cluster – These formations are recognized by the fact that they exhibit many points emerging from the base. Ranging in size from very small to extremely large, each specimen is unique.

Crystal Clusters radiate energy into the area around them and can also be used to absorb negative energies, thereby bringing increased harmony to the life force within the area, be it one's home or place of work.

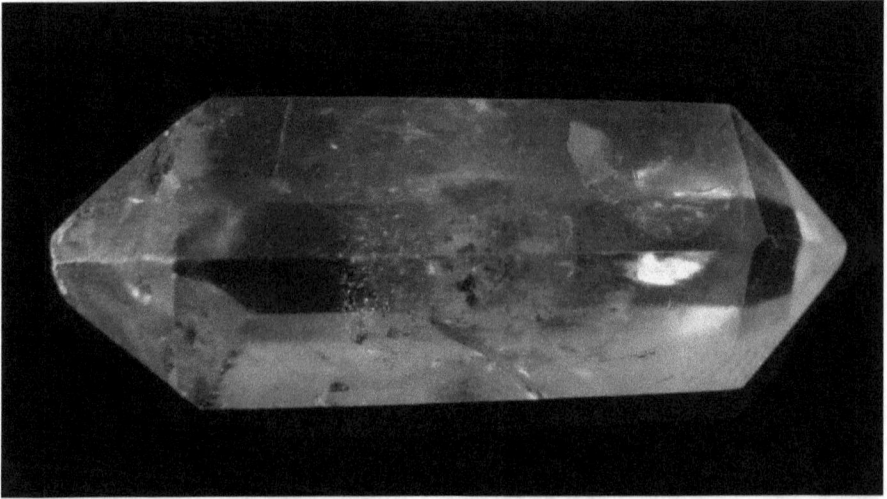

Double Terminated Crystal – As the name suggests, these crystals have a point on each end. They have the capacity to both push and pull energy through their ends. By placing a double terminated crystal in between the chakras, they can then be used to move energy both upwards and downwards through the chakra column of the physical body.

Double Terminated (DT) crystals strengthen energy flow, and are especially useful when you need to share, or exchange, energy between you and another person.

Double Terminated crystals are very important to people doing healing work for themselves or others.

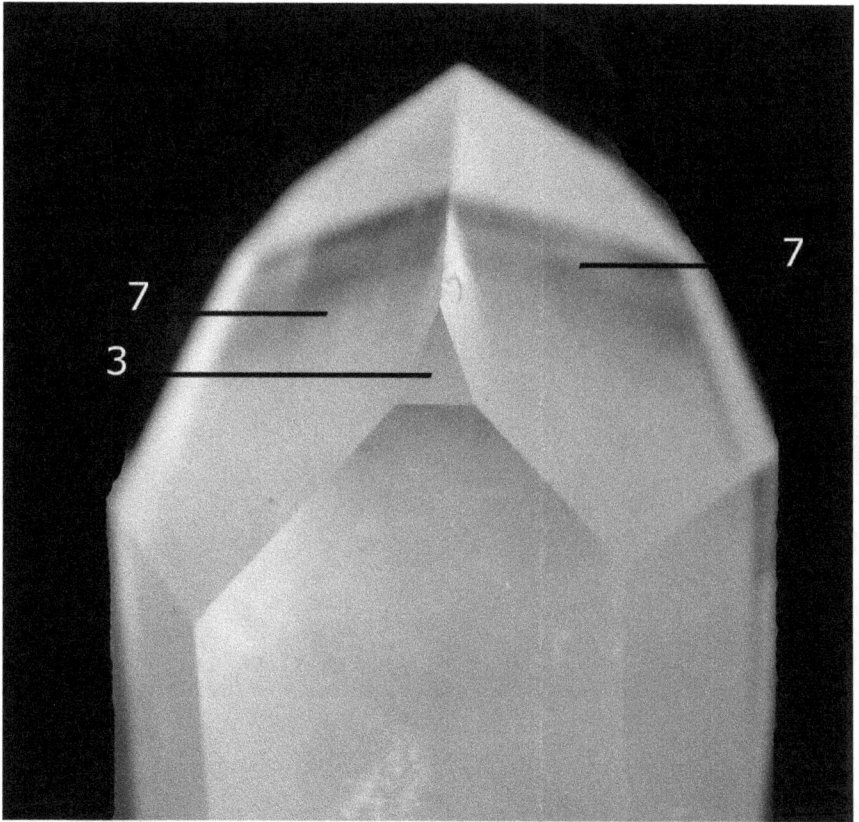

Dow (Trans-Channeling) Crystal – A crystal with three, primary, seven sided faces, with three secondary triangular faces situated in between, giving us a 7 – 3 – 7 – 3 – 7 – 3 configuration. It is believed that this crystal is a combination crystal that incorporates the properties of both a Channnneling and a Transmitter crystal in one formation, helping to facilitate intuitive awareness and connection with the *All That Is*. It is also considered one of the Twelve Master Crystals and is a powerful teaching and healing crystal.

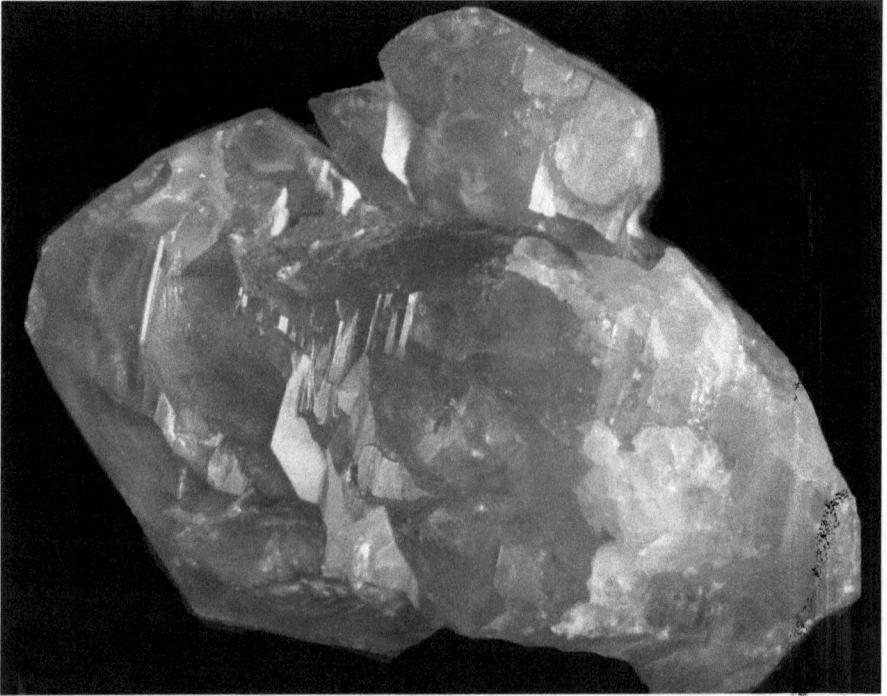

Elestial Quartz Crystal – These truly amazing crystals are easily recognizable by the number of terminations all over them.

Unlike other crystals, Elestials have been formed in water, and this gives them their unique appearance, one that takes on a layered and/or etched effect.

Compared to a complex computer, given their multi-terminations, it is said that Elestial crystals work to bring that which is needed within the grasp of the conscious mind.

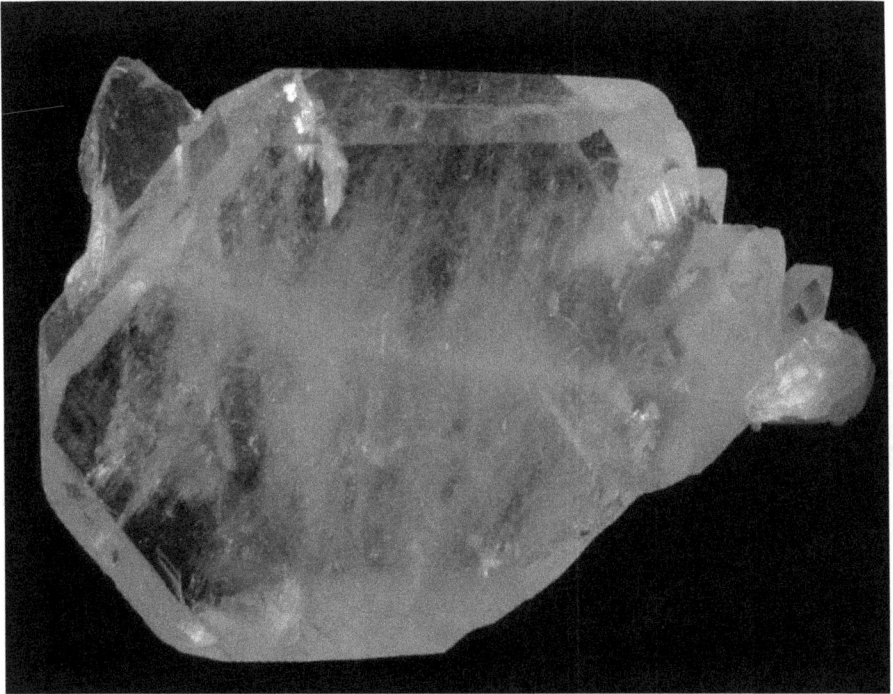

Faden Crystal – These crystals have, clearly visible within their interior structure, a white threadlike line, that runs through the crystal, from one end to the other. These lines are the indicators that Faden crystals were formed in the midst of shifts in the earth surrounding them, causing them to break and later heal.

Understandably, Faden pieces can be used to for healing on all levels, while also providing physical, mental and emotional stability, given that they contain, within their structure, the pattern of their own healing.

It has been stated that this crystal can also be used for both astral travel as well as for assisting us in understanding the lessons we are here to learn in this particular incarnation.

When seeking out information pertinent to one's growth as an individual, Faden crystals are pertinent. Likewise, they also can be used to help balance the physical body.

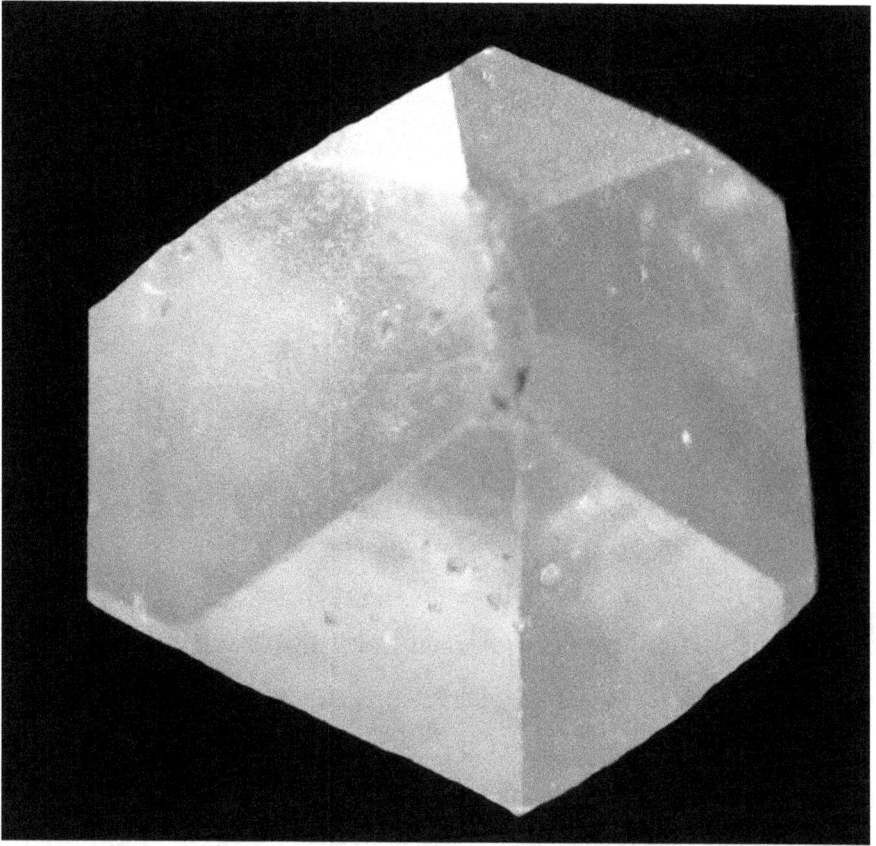

Generator (Merlin) Crystal – A crystal with six evenly spaced sides and six approximately equal faces that center at the tip, coming to a pyramid point, is called a Generator point.

Thought to be a powerful generator of energy, through storing, amplifying and transmitting, this rare crystal has been said that it can act as a connector between like-minded individuals, making it suitable for those who offer group workshops and classes.

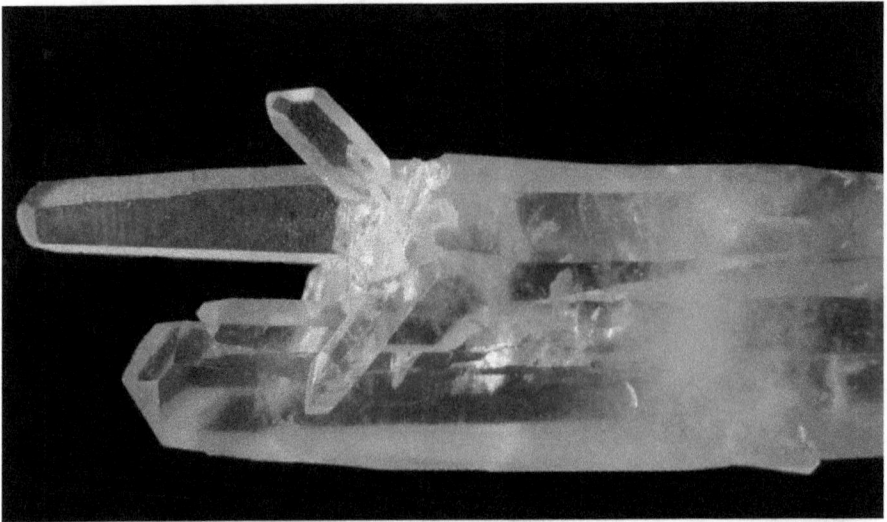

Growth Interference Crystal – A crystal that has various cuts on the body that appears to have been done with a trim saw. Thin, flat calcite crystals have interfered with the growth pattern of the quartz crystal.

While this crystal has been subject to a drastic change of shape, it continues to develop to completion; the key energy signature affiliated with these crystal types.

It is said that Growth Interference crystals are most helpful pieces in overcoming obstacles of every type imaginable, including meditation.

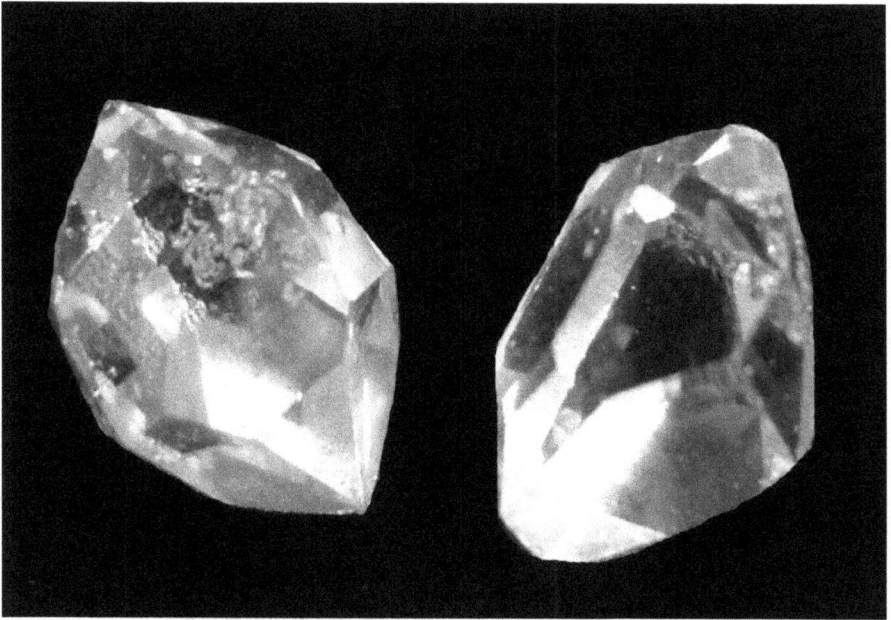

Herkimer Diamond – Herkimer Diamonds are beautiful double-terminated quartz crystals which are found mainly in Herkimer County, New York (USA). Incredibly, these phenomenal gemstones are found in Dolomite rock that has been dated close to five hundred million years old.

The majority of the Herkimer Diamonds have eighteen faces with six triangular faces forming the termination points on each end of the crystal, which are further separated by a group of six square or rectangular faces. It is this particular hexagonal conglomeration that often results in a diamond shape.

Formally discovered in the late 1700's, they often display the sparkling clarity akin to Diamonds; hence the name. The most common mineral on earth … silica … becomes a sparkling little gem in keeping with Herkimer Diamonds.

Amazing amplifiers of energy, Herkimer Diamonds are said to assist with balance on all levels (mental, emotional and physical).

Likewise, they are said to be a master class crystal because they imbue clarity on all levels.

Furthermore, they demonstrate an ability to empower the self, providing the energy to create and manifest visions (mental pictures) into being.

Feel free to refer to the Double Terminated configuration (on page 86) for additional information.

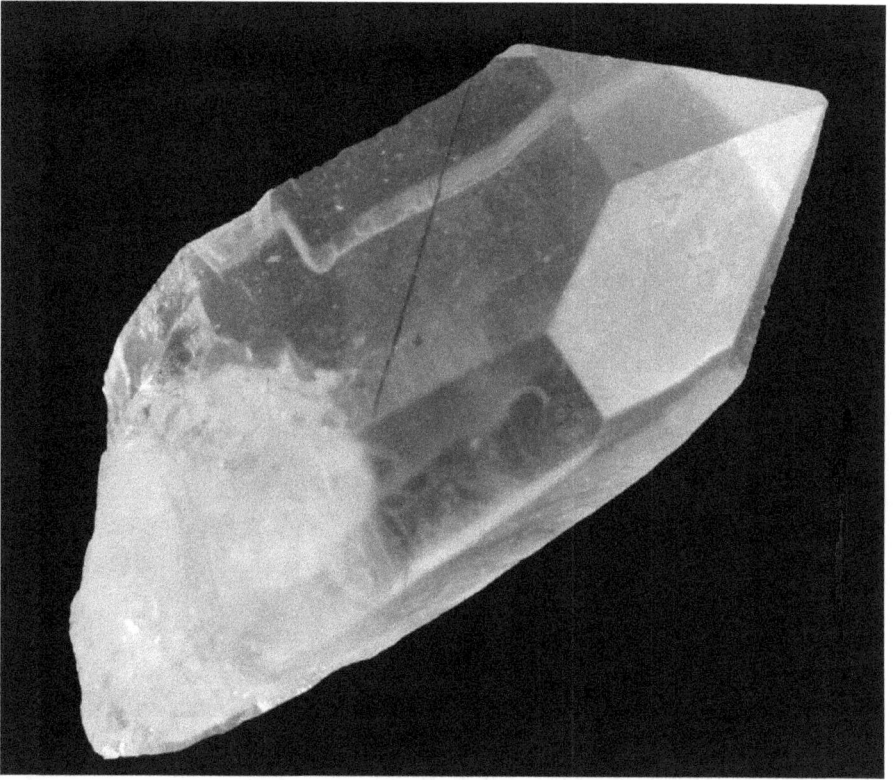

Isis Crystal – A crystal with a relatively symmetrical five sided face is called an Isis crystal.

It is believed the Isis crystal will put you in touch with, and strongly amplify, your feminine energy, thereby assisting you in both acknowledging, and working with, the female or unselfish side of yourself, no matter if you are a man or a woman.

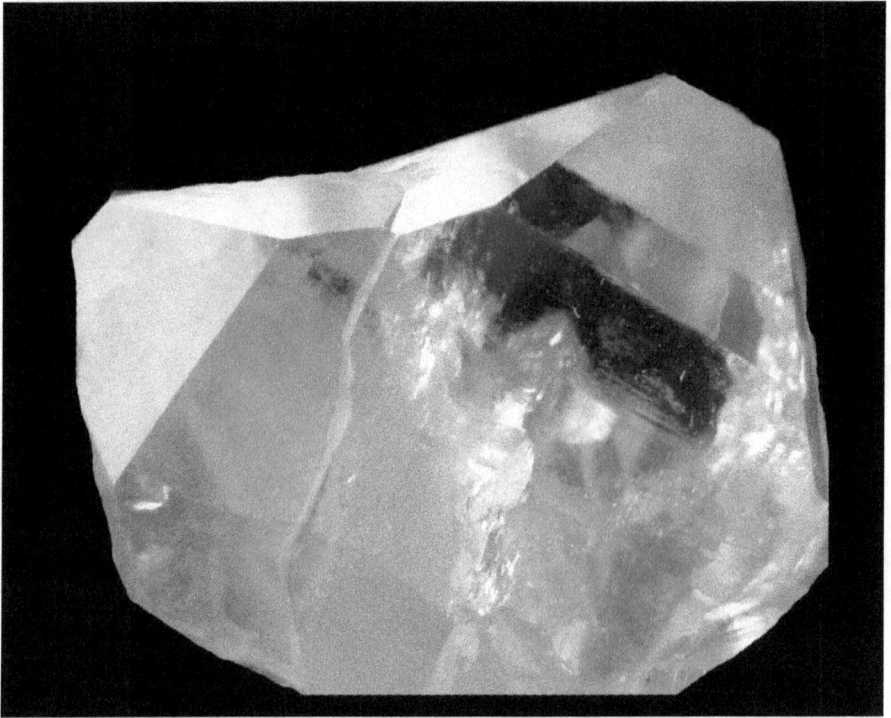

Japanese Law Twin Crystal – The rarest form of twin crystal formation, these configurations are identified as two crystal points cleaving together at approximately 90 degrees. They are found only in a handful of locations around the world, one being Japan.

It has been stated that these crystals can be utilized to clean one's aura, to stabilize one's emotions and to dispel anger. Likewise, this crystal has been used to align the auric body with the physical body (through dissipating and transmuting deviations within the physical body).

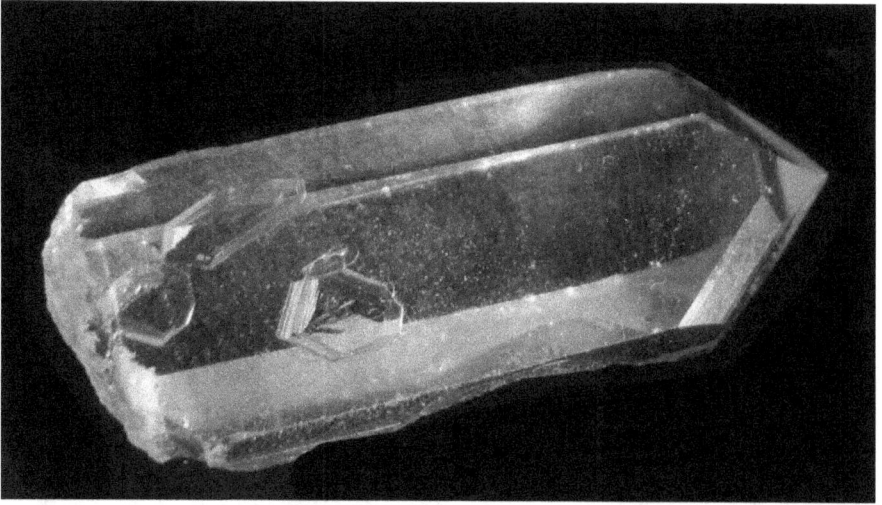

Key Crystal – The Key crystal is recognized by an indentation on the side, or face, of a crystal. The indentation can be either three sided or six sided. As a key unlocks a door, so, too, is it said that these crystals can be used to gain access to information that is normally inaccessible.

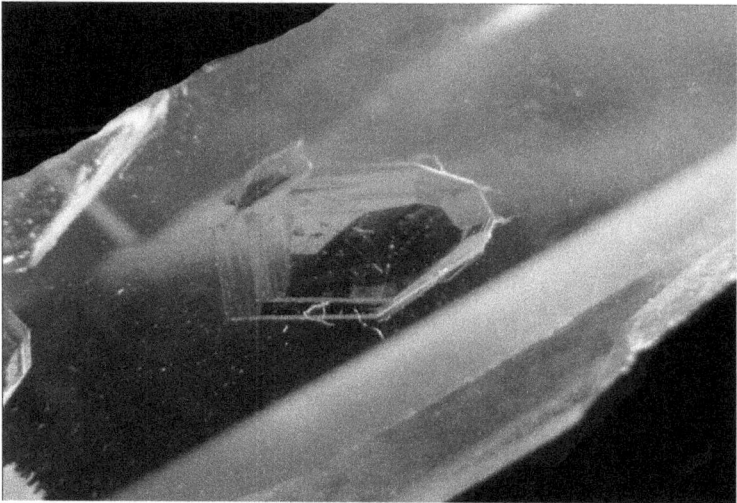

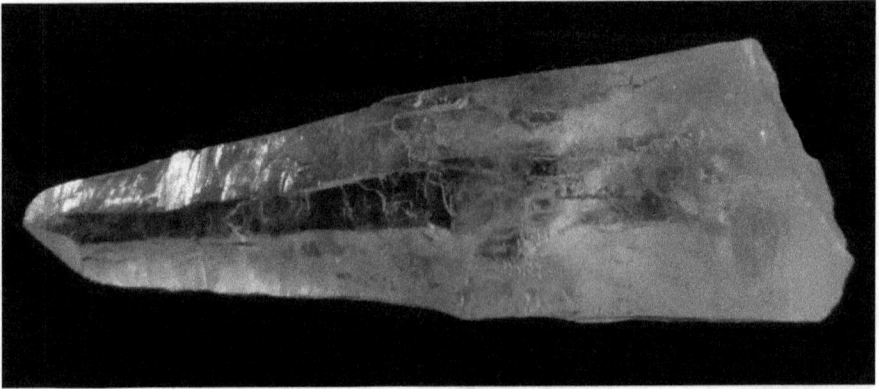

Laser Wand Crystal – Laser crystals are long and slender quartz crystals which are tapered to the termination. They have been said to resemble frozen icicles, for those, like myself, always in need of a visual image.

These crystals are used for many healing purposes, including the ability to clear negative energy from one's light body (aura). They are great tools to use in releasing fear, while allowing one to have the courage to discover their purpose in life.

They can also be used to transmit very concentrated beams of energy into any area where energy is needed.

Laser crystals are also ideal for joining up the crystals within a crystal mandala.

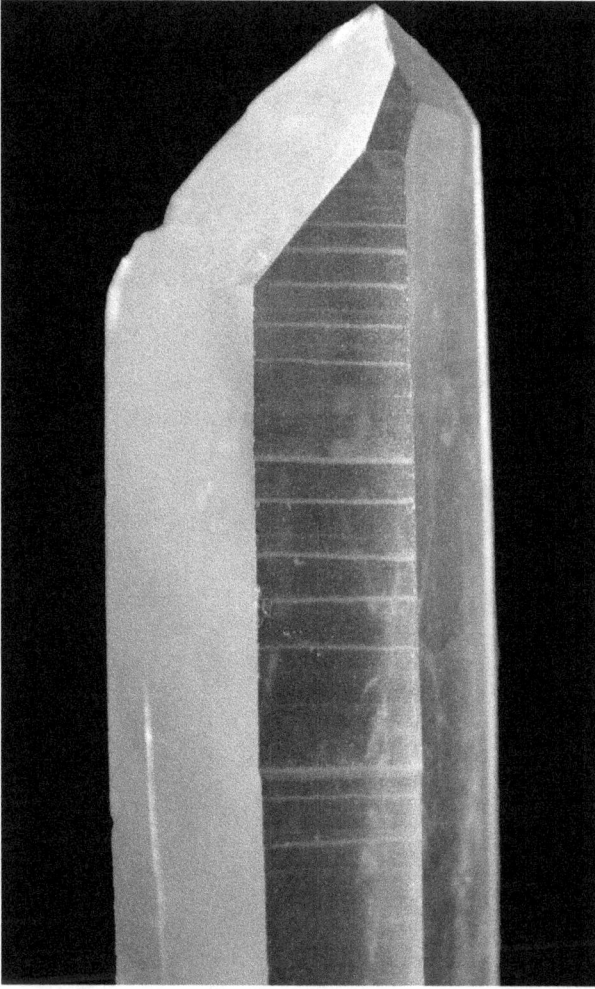

Lemurian Seed Crystal – This crystal configuration is easily recognizable by the horizontal striations running up one or more (usually alternating) sides. They also appear to have a matte surface. Lemurian Seed Crystals are reputed to have been left by the Lemurians, an advanced ancient civilization, to teach and guide us in this time. These crystals have been programmed with conscious connection and love.

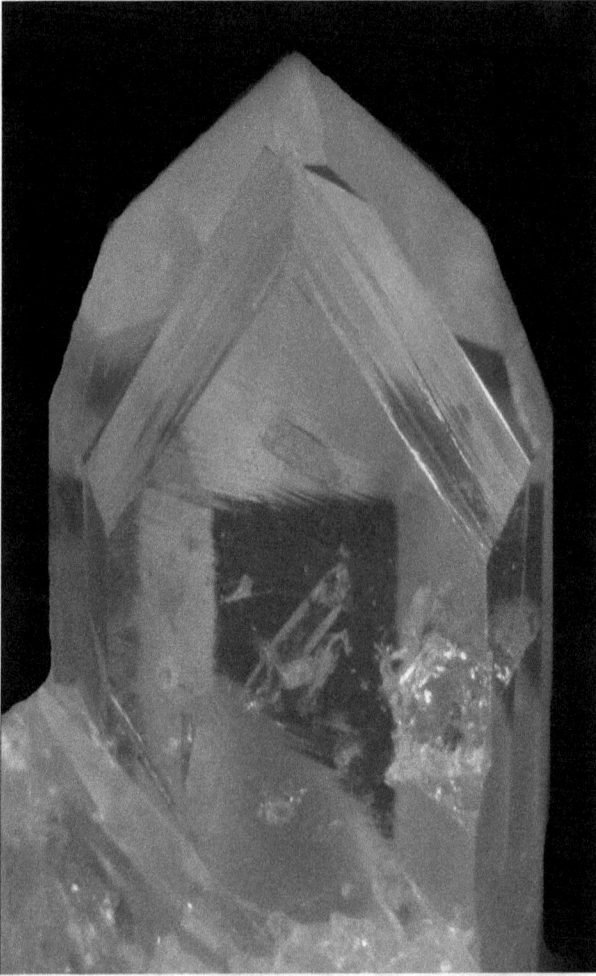

Lineated Crystal – These crystals are characterized by their parallel raised or rectilinear indented lines. These lines were not etched into the crystal; rather, they were caused by the growth against another pattern configuration. Used extensively by the Native Americans in their vision quests, these crystals provide a connection between the physical realm and the vision realm.

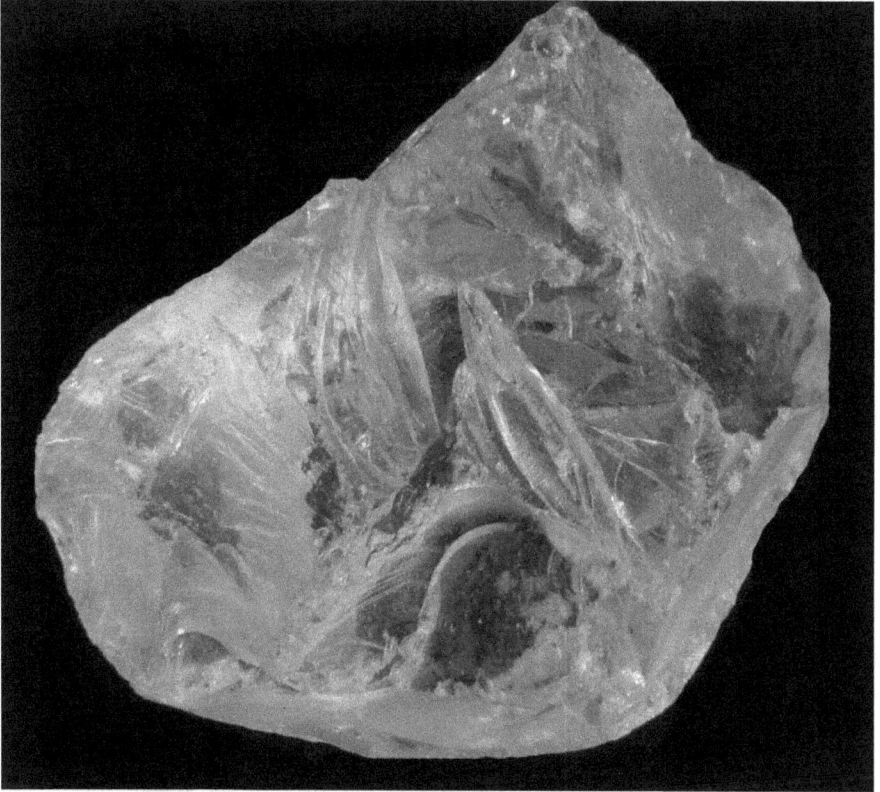

Optical Crystal – The name of this crystal configuration specifically refers to the high level of purity, clarity and luster rarely found in natural Quartz crystals.

This intense crystal enables one to look within, to delve into the unknown, all in an effort to discover why we are here at this time.

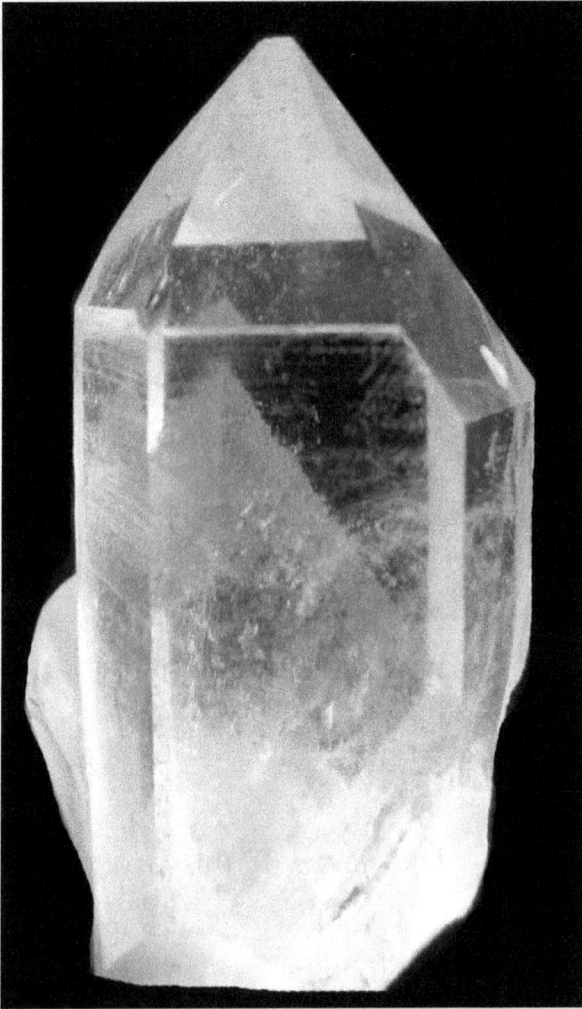

Phantom and Included Quartz – These formations are reasonably rare, but they can be found with all types of phantoms in them, containing different types of minerals.

The phantom is caused by a pause in the growth of the crystal (which can last for thousands of years).

As the crystal resumes its growth, the phantom remains within the crystal.

Phantom crystals have a tendency to come into your life at a time when you are carrying an immense amount of pain. Knowing that these crystals can assist one in the healing of their emotional injuries, it becomes quite fitting if you find yourself spending time with one.

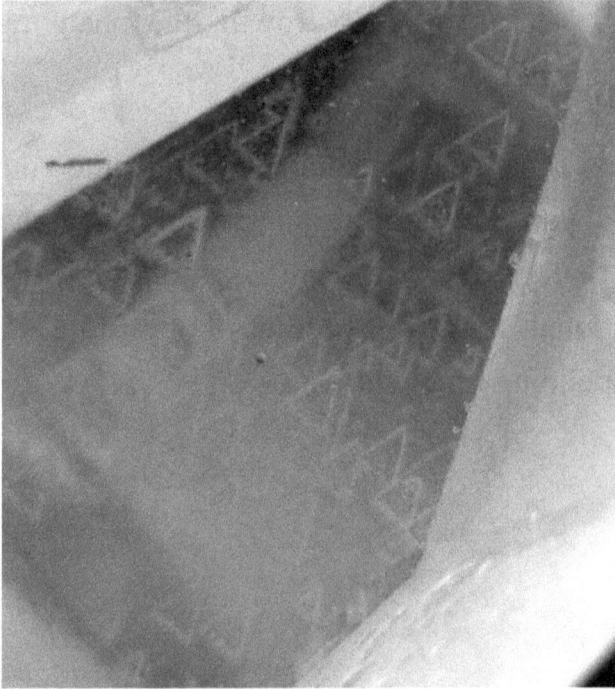

Record Keeper Crystal – These crystals have a raised pyramid, or triangle on one face. You may also discover many of these distinctive markings on several faces of the crystal.

Carefully check all the faces of any quartz crystals that come into your possession. Sometimes you will need to reflect a light source off the faces, in order to be able to clearly see the triangular markings.

It is not only Quartz that can be Record Keepers.

These crystals are said to hold information that was recorded there thousands of years ago, from the times of Lemuria and Atlantis.

Libraries of stored information, meditating with them will allow you to access their information. You can also activate them by rubbing your thumb across the pyramidal triangles, in the same way that you can activate Tabular crystals by rubbing your thumbnail over the lines that are ingrained upon them.

It is believed that the Record Keeper is one of the most sacred crystals because it holds the wisdom and knowledge of the universe.

When a person is properly attuned to a Record Keeper, this ancient knowledge (which contains profound secrets and esoteric knowledge of the whole of the Higher consciousness) is readily made available.

Understandably, it takes both an open mind as well as a pure heart to access this knowledge.

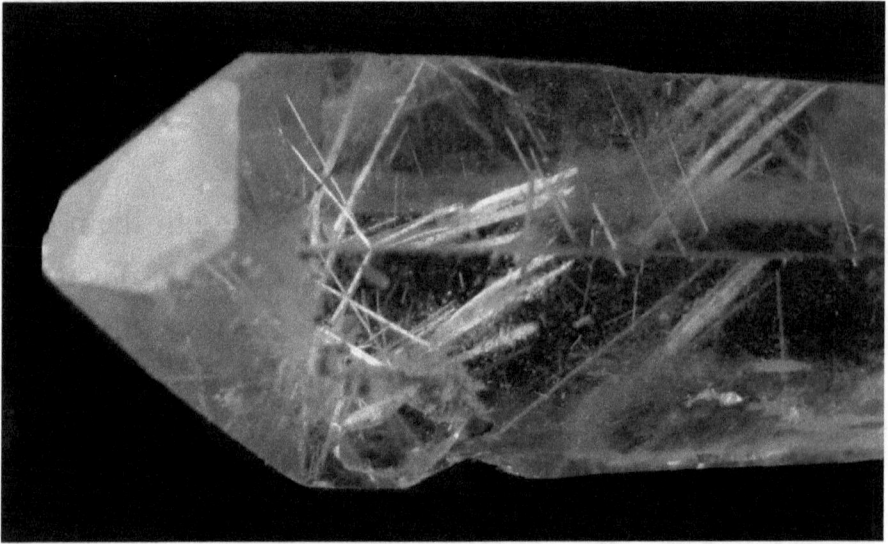

Rutile Inclusion Crystal – These crystals are easily recognizable by their inclusion of rutile (tiny straight threads or needle like crystals of titanium dioxide), said to enhance the metaphysical properties of its host crystal.

Since Quartz is already a very strong and versatile piece, this combination really provides one with a powerful tool for spiritual and self-healing purposes.

Rutilated Quartz can assist you by clearing away negative energy and energy blockages, thereby magnifying, and enhancing, all positive energy entering your auric system.

This is an immensely beautiful crystal that must be seen and experienced by the individual.

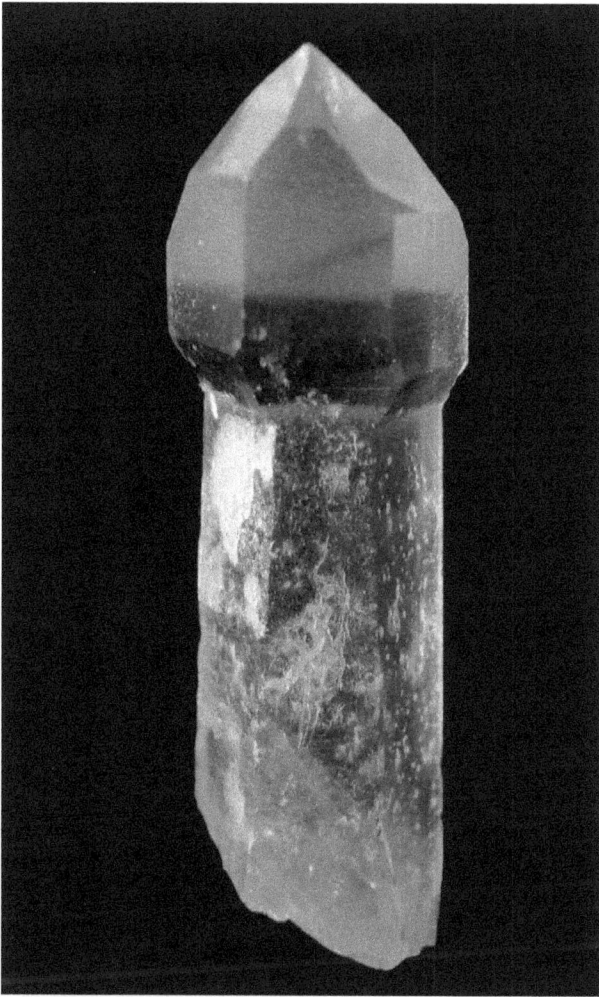

Scepter Crystal – These crystals, which are recognized by a long, thin, crystal rod, have another crystal growing around the tip. In actuality, the crystal on the top (that which appears to be the tip), later formed around the rod.

It is popularly believed that such crystals were used by the priests and priestesses of Lemuria and Atlantis.

Scepter Cystals bring the spirituality of the higher planes into ceremonies of a healing nature, focusing the energy deep within the heart of the matter.

This particular configuration is also excellent for the transmission of directional energy.

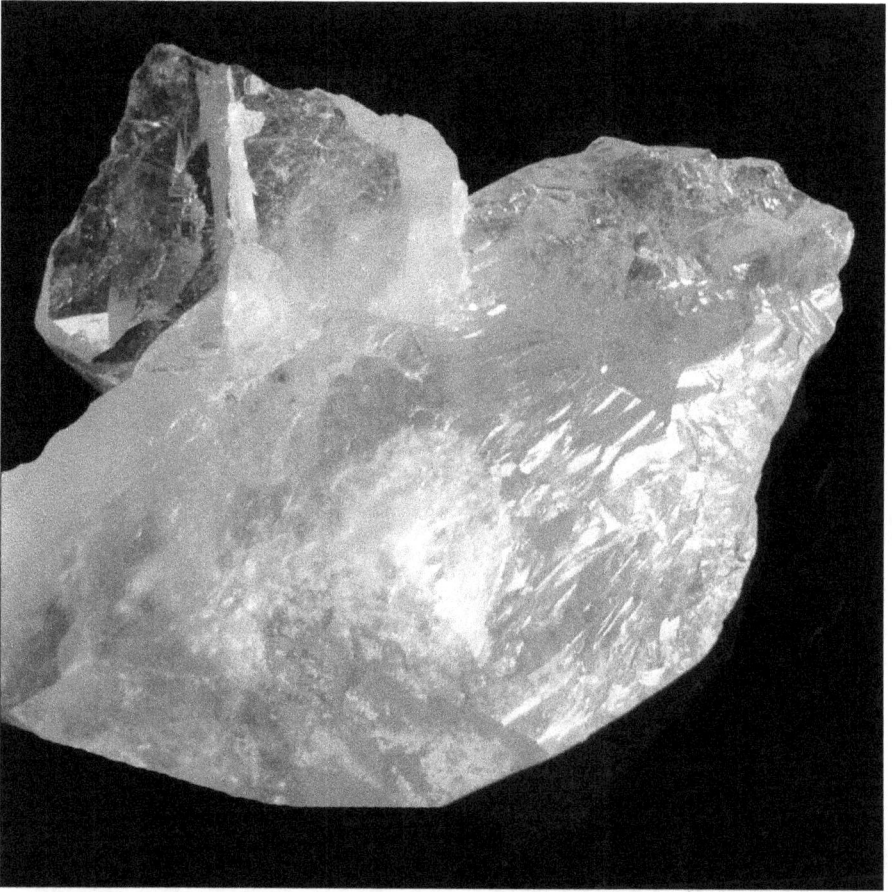

Self-Healed (Shard) Crystal – These crystals are recognized by crystalline structures appearing where a crystal was previously broken. The ultimate form of self-healing, these crystals are very important to us as healing facilitators.

It is believed that these crystals can be used as a guide to one's own self-healing journey, be it physical, emotional, mental, or spiritual.

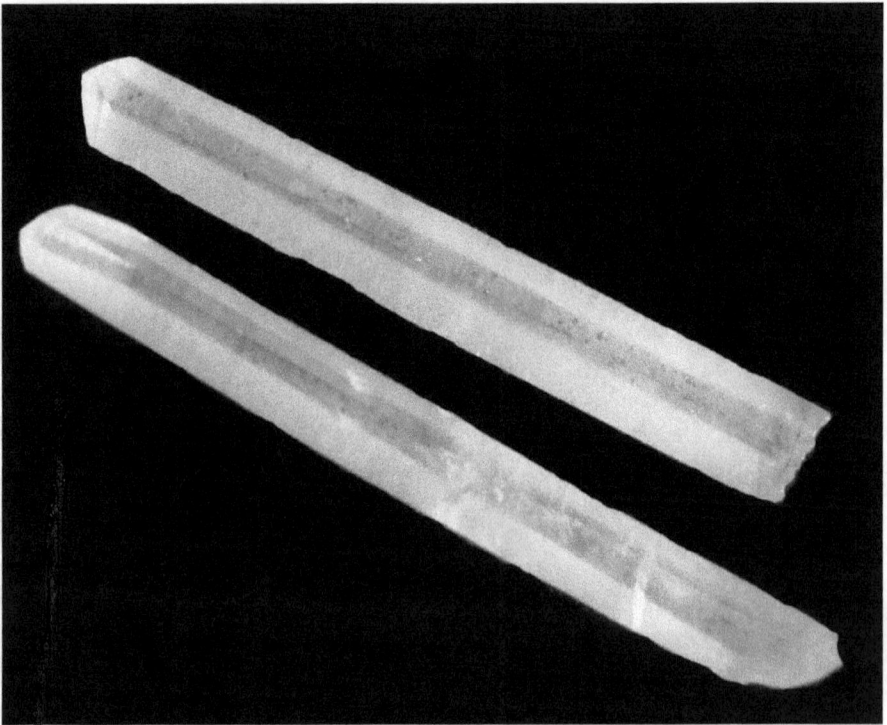

Singing Crystals – These quartz crystals pieces, usually long and thin, make a high pitched singing sound when gently rubbed or rolled together.

Said to contain a powerful OM vibration, they are most useful in generating creative energies. A rare configuration, they are known to come from Brazil.

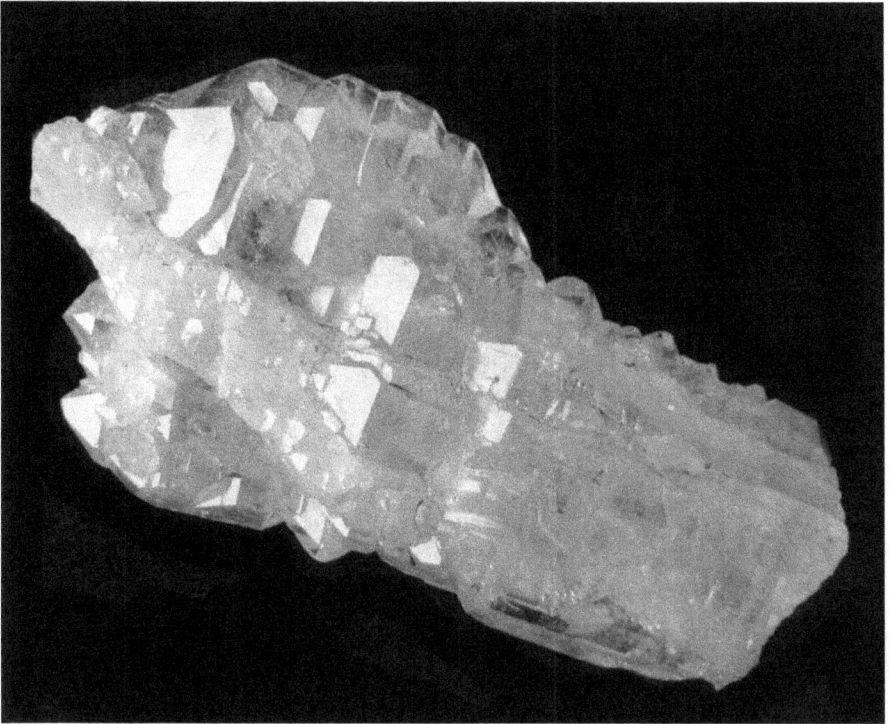

Skeletal Crystal – This particular formation often displays unusual surface patterns and curved distortions of the faces. While they might look like fractures, they are actually growth forms.

This very important and highly unique crystal has been known to assist individuals who are experiencing significantly rough times, helping them to better understand the experience while also offering ideas (which may, in certain circumstances, be seen as solutions) that allow them to work through the difficulty.

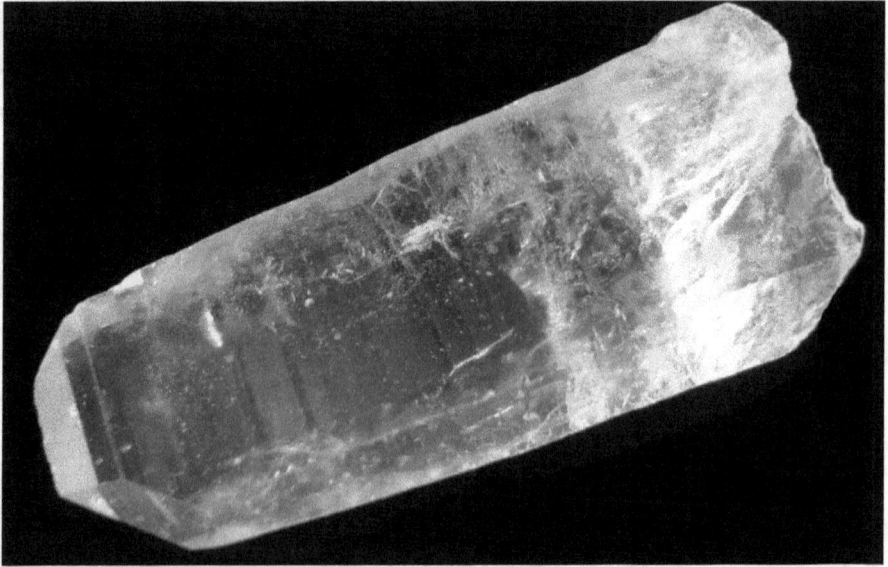

Tabular (Tabby) Crystal – A crystal with a flattened tabular shape, whereby two of its opposite sides are twice as wide, or more, than its other sides, giving the overall appearance of a tablet, is called a Tabular crystal.

These crystals are said to enhance communication, while also smoothing the energy flow, as a means of integrating both ideas and balance.

In this way, they facilitate understanding and dialogue between people.

They can also help us communicate, in a more authentic manner, with nature.

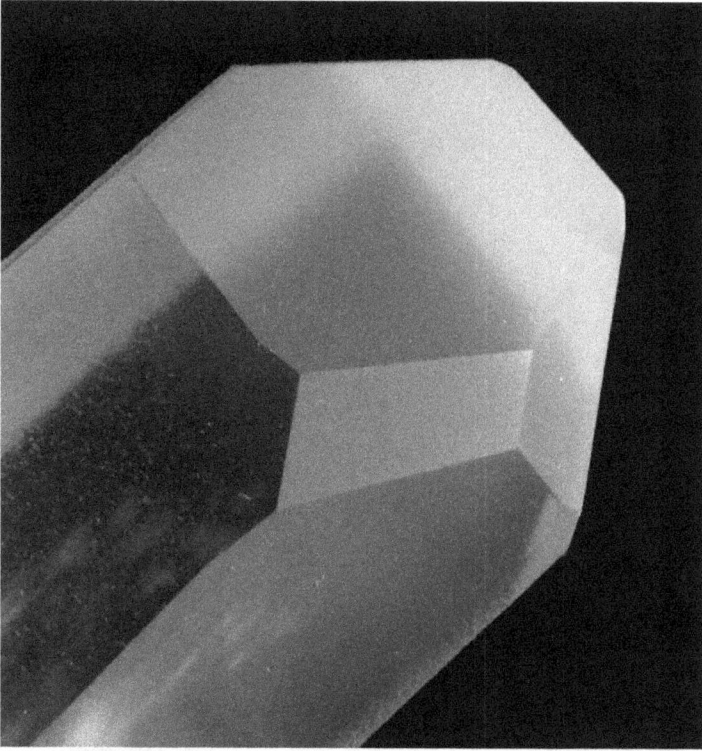

Time Line to the Future Crystal – These right activation crystals are recognized by having an inclined window that leans to the right hand side of the front of the crystal.

It is believed they can be used to access information from the future. It is also said that right activation crystals increase right brain functions such as visuals, seeing patterns and intuition.

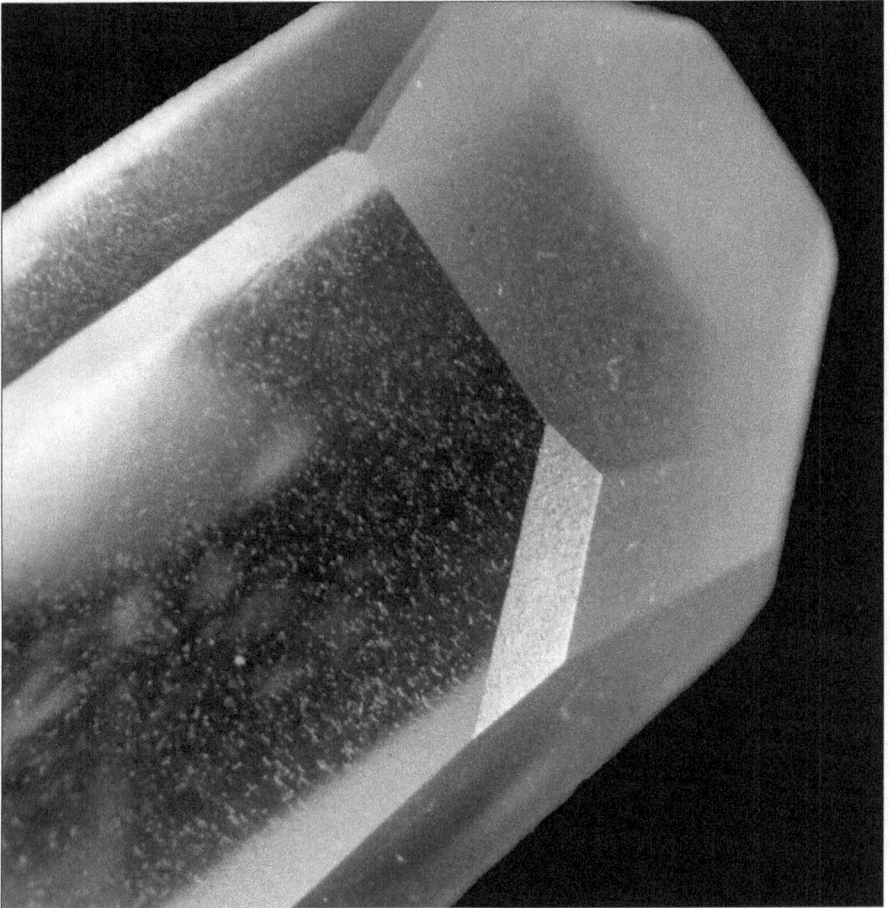

Time Line to the Past Crystal – These left activation crystals are recognized by having an inclined window that leans to the left hand side of the front of the crystal. It is believed they can be used to access information from the past. It is also said that left activation crystals increase left brain functions such as analysis, objectivity, rationality, verbal skills, logic and planning.

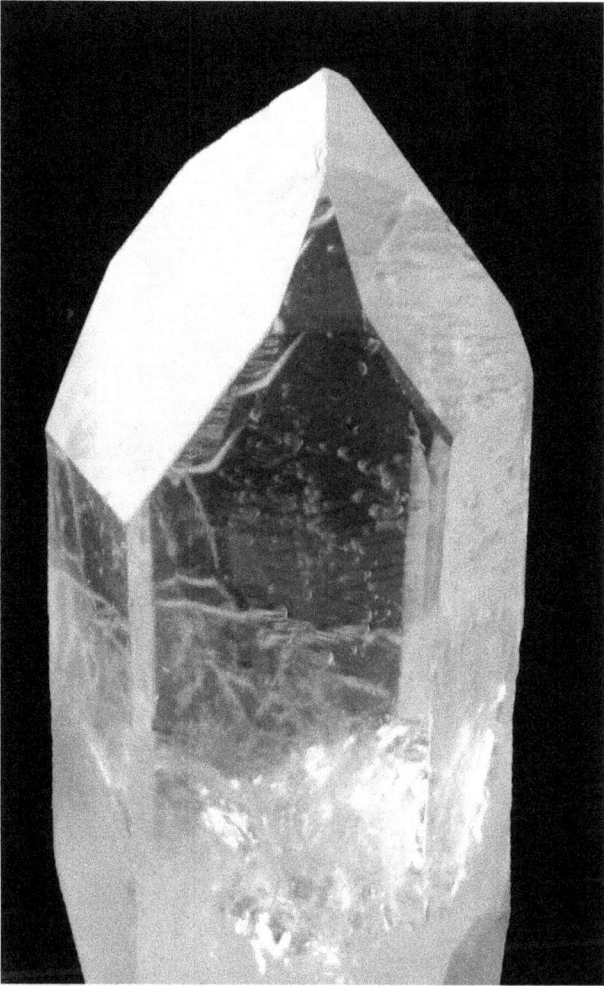

Transmitter Crystal – A crystal with two, seven sided faces, and a single perfect triangular face situated in between, giving us a 7 – 3 – 7 configuration. Transmitter crystals, it is said, can be used to help connect one to higher wisdom, including their higher (subconscious) self. They are excellent for helping to find answers to puzzling questions.

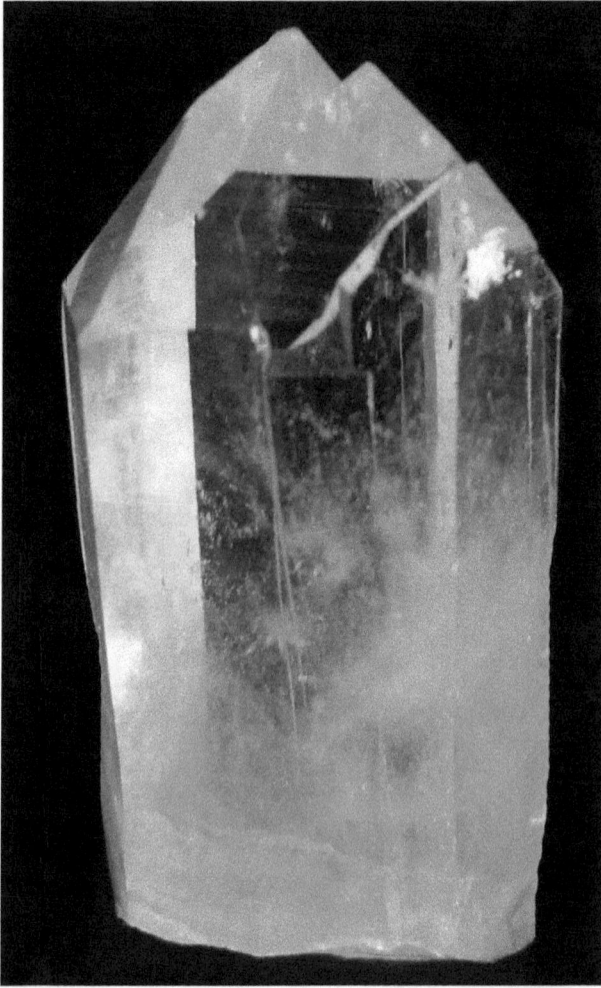

Triple Crystal – The three separately formed terminations at the point make this a highly desirable crystal for connecting family members. Likewise, this crystal can also offer information to parents, so that they, too, may connect with their children, bringing happy and fun energy into the home.

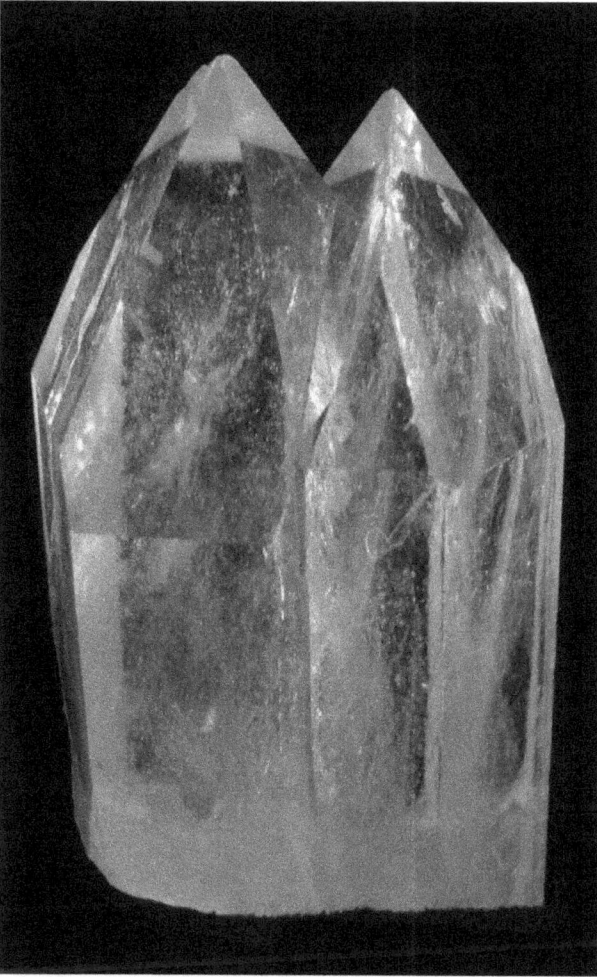

Twin Crystal (also known as Tantric Twin) – A crystal with two points on a common base is called a twin crystal. You can tell a twin crystal from two crystals that are simply attached to each other, by the fact that both parts of a twin crystal are exactly parallel to each other, and have no boundary between them.

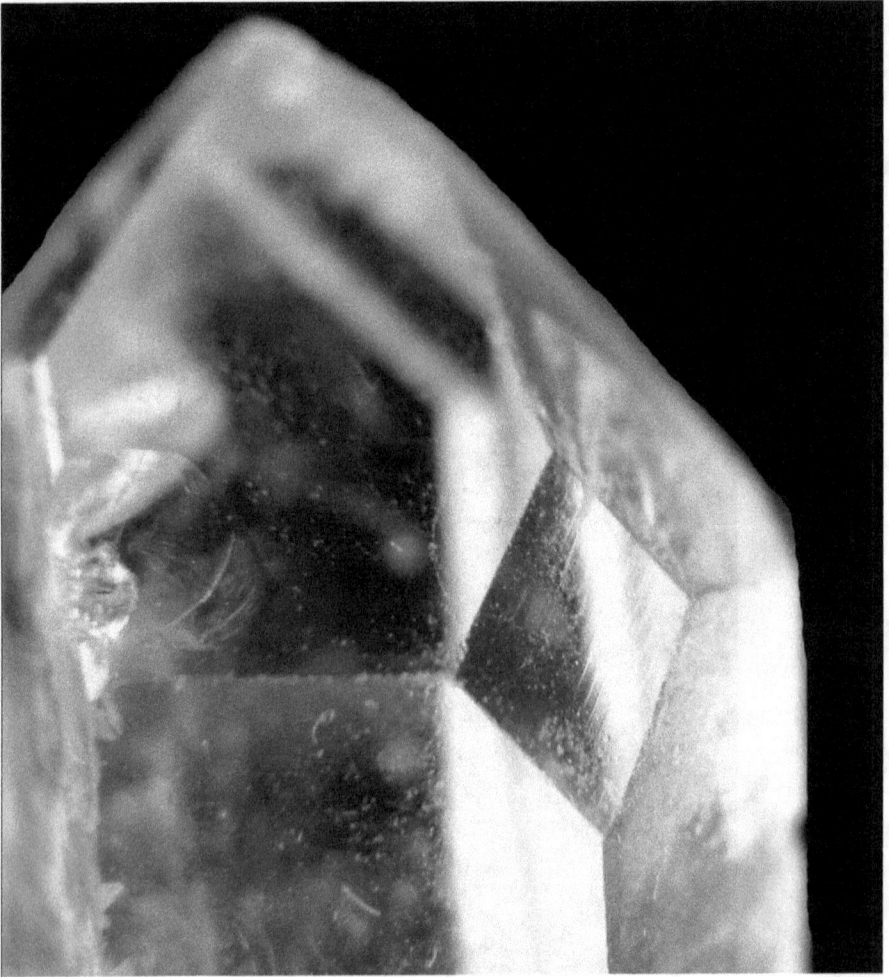

Window Crystal – These crystals have a diamond or rectangular face between the body and tip of a point that is called a window. It is believed that this crystal will open a window to your soul and help you get intuitive answers to questions through bypassing the conscious mind (ego).

Manifestation Crystal – A crystal with a small crystal totally enclosed within a larger crystal is a called a Manifestation crystal. From a geometric point of view, these crystals can be viewed as a *world within a world*.

Rainbow Crystal – A crystal with an inside rainbow, one that is caused by light being refracted by the prismatic effect of a crack or inclusion. It is believed that these crystals exhibit the closest manifestation of pure white light that can be witnessed on the physical plane.

Yin and Yang Clarity Crystal – The first impression of quality or value of natural crystal is usually judged by the clarity. The clarity ranges from milky white to glass clear that sparkles like a cut diamond.

The *milky white* crystal is said to represent the yin or feminine qualities of love, communication, negotiation and receptivity.

The *clear* crystal represents the yang or masculine qualities of power, force, strength and creativity.

A crystal with both is believed to promote a balance of the masculine and feminine energy on both physical and mental levels.

A belief or belief system is a filter used by consciousness to create an experience or to judge what has not been personally experienced. Beliefs or belief systems will focus our attention either on what we want or what we do not want, thereby creating the reality we perceive.

Imagine discovering a very clear, shiny rock with six smooth sides and terminated with a sharp point. No human being could have made this. Natural quartz crystal has evoked many questions because of the unknowns about its origin and purpose.

To explain the unknowns, human beings imagined all kinds of possibilities that evolved into beliefs. Because of the beauty, it was only natural to assign sacred or spiritual significance to crystal.

American Indians, Tibetan monks, Druid priests and many other groups, proclaimed the sacred power of crystal. Because they believed in the sacred power or spiritual significance of crystal, evidence was manifested to support their beliefs. These beliefs worked for them and the evidence was positive and good.

Today, many people use crystals to help focus their attention on something they want or to align with, and access, information from a higher level of consciousness.

Many unique geometric configurations and characteristics of quartz crystal have been labelled with special names. Books have been written by practitioners that detail the use and expected results of these special crystals.

Since the information is not always in agreement, the reader is left to decide what feels right or to dismiss the whole concept and merely appreciate the natural beauty of crystal.

Most all the beliefs about quartz crystal involve its energy properties.

The most common or universal belief system involves the scientific use of both natural and synthetic crystals in optics, acoustics and electronic applications. If you watch TV or use a computer, you have to believe in this application. With a little imagination you can explore the following beliefs about unique geometric configurations and characteristics of natural quartz crystals.

No matter what we believe or want to believe, we cannot deny the inherent beauty of natural quartz crystal.

Even more amazing is that, like crystal, every human being has the same natural beauty if they will let it shine or if we take the time to look for it.

Just as our beliefs about crystal create what we experience with them, our judgment of other human beings has the power to either create separation or integration. Since we each have a free will and a choice in what we believe, we should focus our attention on what we want rather than on the things we do not want. If crystal will help us do this, then it becomes a valuable tool in life.

If you are attracted to crystal and appreciate the beauty, then know that what you see in a crystal is merely a reflection of who you really are. By daring to let the real you shine for others to enjoy and appreciate, you will add to the natural beauty of our planet.

Copyright © Stuart Schmitt [29]

Reprinted with permission.

---

[29] http://www.arcrystalmine.com/index.php

Each type of stone gives off its own unique form of subtle energy. The particular energy given off by a stone is determined by its internal crystalline structure, and by the atomic vibrations that are specific to that structure.

Certain stones, including most of the stones normally thought of as healing stones, vibrate in a way that resonates with and strengthens particular energies inside each person. These are the energies of the inner self, the energies that make up the attitudes and human qualities of a person.

This resonance can occur because the inner self operates by using a type of subtle energy that is similar to the subtle energy of crystals and stones.

The reason this type of energy is called "subtle energy" is because, although it is physical, it is less physical in nature than normal types of energy such as heat, electricity or mechanical energy.

Subtle energy is what puts the "meta" in metaphysical. It is subtle because it is hard to measure.

Science has not figured out how to measure it yet, and what science cannot measure, it does not believe in.

In spite of its many great achievements, science would not even know where to begin to measure your personal energy in order to find out how much subtle energy you are putting out in the form of human qualities such as patience or acceptance at any given time.

Because of its somewhat less physical nature, subtle energy reveals itself in a quieter, often slower and more gentle, way than the more physical types of energy.

For example, if you put a stone or quartz crystal in your pocket and carry it around with you, it may take some time, perhaps a day, before you notice the effect from it.

THE DIFFERENCE BETWEEN CRYSTALS AND STONES

Both quartz crystals and certain types of stones strengthen the energies of the inner self, but each does it in a slightly different way.

A stone gives off a very specific narrow (in bandwidth) type of subtle energy vibration because of its crystalline structure and chemical makeup, and it is the stone itself that is the source of this vibration.

In contrast, quartz crystals are called the "master stone" because they operate in a much broader way that amplifies all the subtle energy frequencies.

This happens because quartz crystals, unlike stones, are not the actual source of the subtle energy vibration, but instead they amplify, and then reflect back, those subtle energy vibrations that exist in their immediate environment. For this reason, a quartz crystal is able to strengthen all the energies of the inner self at once.

For example, if you feel loving toward someone, and you are carrying a quartz crystal in your pocket at the time, that crystal will amplify and intensity the love energy you put out by resonating with it and making it stronger.

Although stones and quartz crystals operate somewhat differently, each has its purpose. It only works in its own specific area, that is, each stone only strengthens the particular energy or human quality it resonates with.

This makes stones ideal for concentrating on your growth by working on one energy at a time, or working on several energies at once by using several stones.

Because of its broad and more general way of operating, a quartz crystal works to strengthen all areas of the inner self at the same time.

Because a quartz crystal strengthens everything at once, it does not usually change the balance of the energies, and balance in the energies is extremely important, sometimes even more important than growth itself.

This is why stones are important. They cannot only strengthen the energies, but, if chosen properly, they can bring the weaker energies up closer in strength to the stronger energies, and produce an internal balance that gives you a serenity and peacefulness that comes from being of one mind (not of divided opinion) in all areas of your life.

THE EFFECTS OF DISTANCE

The effect that stones and crystals have on the inner self falls off with distance. The larger a stone is, the more energy it puts out, and the farther that energy radiates from it. Although a small stone vibrates in the same way as a large stone of the same type, it affects a smaller area with its energy than a large stone.

For example, if you wear a small quartz crystal around your neck, it essentially puts out personal energy, in that the energy does not affect others much, but stays close to you. Its sphere of influence is just around you, with an effective radius of about one foot.

Hand held crystals of about ¾ inch diameter have a larger sphere of influence, with an effective radius of perhaps 2 to 4 feet.

A three inch diameter crystal will fill a large room or small apartment with energy that will have a positive impact on everyone in that area.

CRYSTALS, STONES AND PERSONAL GROWTH

By themselves, crystals and stones do not make you a better person or a different person from what you are. But they *do* resonate with the subtle energy of your inner self, your attitudes or human qualities, to make them stronger and more intense, so it becomes more obvious to you what is going on inside.

This makes it easier for you to see who you are and what you want to change about yourself in order to become a better person.

But keep in mind that your attitudes do not change unless you want them to, and that you are the one responsible for any growth you do.

A stone can only amplify an aspect of who you already are. To grow as a person, you must do the work yourself.

Crystals and stones can be of really good help in personal growth, but keep in mind that they are not magic.

What they do is give you an edge in growth because of how the vibrations of their crystalline structure interact with the inner self.

Crystals and stones have the ability to resonate with the different energies of the inner self, thereby strengthening those energies. This additional strength gives you the internal boost your energies need to make it easier to take steps towards growth.

It gives you the extra insight and determination you need to take the leap of faith that is necessary in adopting a new attitude. It also gives you the strength to not be afraid to change something about yourself. But in spite of all this, you must still do the actual learning and growing.

The magical qualities of crystals and stones lies in the effect they have on people. Because of how they work, crystals and stones have the ability to make someone feel more positive, feeling better about life.

Among other things, the way they interact with a person's inner self enhances the human qualities of loving and caring, which are often considered rather magical in themselves.

Crystals and stones are really considered magical only because they enhance the magic that already exists in people's lives.

Copyright © John and Micki Baumann [30]

Reprinted with permission.

---

[30] http://www.lovesedona.com/

HOW CRYSTALS GROW

Generally, quartz crystals grow in a hexagonal (six sided) structure, with additional faces sloping towards a point at one end. A crystal with these characteristics is itself also called a point. Points may be totally clear and transparent, or they may contain streaks, lines, rainbows, water bubbles or other inclusions. They may also appear cloudy if they have grown in a place where it freezes in the winter. Optical clarity usually has little to do with a crystal's quality and its ability to amplify the subtle energies.

WHAT CRYSTALS DO

Quartz crystals are a gift from the earth. They have the ability to amplify or strengthen the things in you that are positive, and can help you put away things that cause you fear or anger. They can strengthen your ability to be a loving person, and can enhance your abilities to enjoy life and accomplish the things you want in life. They can amplify intention, reduce stress, help with centering (balancing or calming), strengthen healing abilities, and surround you with protection by amplifying white light.

Any healthy quartz crystal point can strengthen these things and help produce personal growth by amplifying the subtle energies that flow inside you.

SELECTING A CRYSTAL

To select a crystal, first put yourself in a calm space. Hold the crystal in your right hand with the point towards you. Feel it physically. Be open to sensations like tingling or a change in the temperature. Feel the crystal emotionally. Think of the purpose you want it for, and see if you feel attracted to it. Be more concerned with how it feels than how it looks. Allow the crystal to pick you by interacting with it in this way. And remember to do this with your initial feeling. If you need a specialized type of crystal to work with, consider one of the types that follow.

THE MOST USUAL FORM OF QUARTZ CRYSTAL

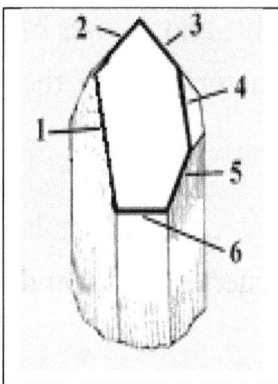

Quartz crystals exist in a number of varieties. In particular, some forms of quartz have different numbers of edges surrounding the largest of the faces that slopes toward the point. A quartz crystal with six edges on the largest face (as shown here) is the most usual type.

It acts as a comprehensive amplifier of the energy in that it strengthens all of a person's energies or human qualities. Its attributes are the most general because it does not have the more specific characteristics of the Isis, Channeling or Grounding crystals that are described herein, which have five, seven or eight edges.

IDENTIFYING SPECIAL PROPERTIES IN QUARTZ CRYSTALS

In addition to the general characteristics mentioned above, quartz crystals sometimes have other special attributes that enhance their power. To identify these special types of crystals, pay particular attention to the largest of the faces that slope toward the point.

Does it have pyramids (triangles) on it?

Count the number of edges surrounding the face. This number can be anywhere from three to eight, and is one of the things that determines the special characteristics of the crystal.

In addition to strengthening the Inner Beings as all crystals do, the listed crystals which follow are true teachers and provide additional special help.

Most of them are relatively rare, and they should be highly treasured when one of them finds you.

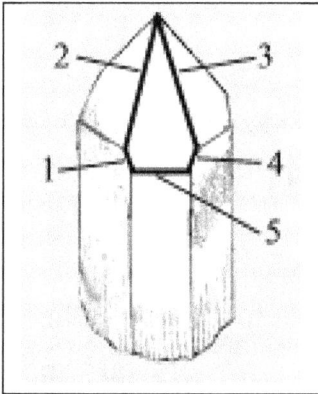

Isis Crystals have five edges surrounding the largest sloping face. These crystals strongly amplify the feminine energy, and can help you get in touch with the "female" or unselfish side of yourself, no matter whether you are a man or a woman.

These crystals are useful in balancing your male-female energy if the female energy has been suppressed, or if you need a greater balance of female energy for any reason. Isis Crystals put you in touch with the power of the Goddess.

For men, the Isis Crystal will help you become more in tune with your feminine side and to become more aware of the aspects of women that you may find troubling.

For women, the Isis Crystal will help you regain some of the power and energy that society has taken from you. It teaches that to be feminine is not weak. Anyone doing healing work with another person needs the Isis energy to be effective.

The Isis Crystal should be carried or held when dealing with issues that are emotional and difficult.

Exercise

Isis Crystals can be used to project nurturing energy toward another person. To do this, sit quietly with the Isis Crystal in your hand with the point directed away from you.

Visualize the person that you wish to help and visualize white light going from the point of the crystal and surrounding the person.

To nurture yourself, sit with the Isis Crystal in your hand with the point directed toward you. Visualize white light going from the point of the crystal and surrounding you. After doing this you should feel strong and cared for.

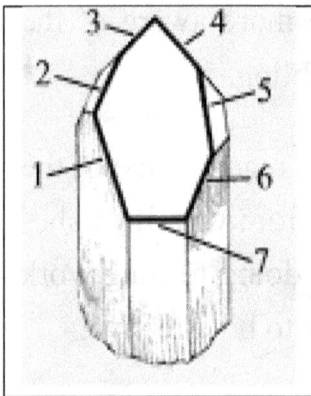

3 4 2 5 1 6 7	Channeling Crystals have seven edges surrounding the largest sloping face. These crystals are especially useful for obtaining information from deep within yourself or from sources that are outside of your normal realm.

They can help you draw on the knowledge and information that is provided by the universe, and can aid you in getting help from a higher source.

A Channeling Crystal can be used anytime you are seeking answers or help from outside yourself. You must "listen" very carefully when using this crystal and realize that answers can come from many sources.

Communication with Guide

A Channeling Crystal is a line of communication with sources outside yourself. Generally, the main source is your guide (a non-physical entity whose primary job is to look after you). Every human has a guide. Guides are sometimes called other things, such as conscience, or angels, but they are always with us. We must learn to listen to what they have to say. Your guide will never tell you what to do, or interfere in other ways with what you do not want to do, but your guide is there to help you find answers for yourself. And you can use your Channeling Crystal to *let your guide be your conscience*.

A Channeling Crystal can only be used by the person holding it. In other words, you cannot send the energy to someone else in order to let him/her receive the information directly.

However, since guides communicate readily with each other, you can become good at getting information to people by asking your guide to give the needed information for someone else, and then relaying it to the person. This is channeling information for others.

Channeling Crystals amplify the quiet inner voice of your guide, and can be a big help in learning how to channel information, both for yourself and for others.

Exercise

Sit quietly holding the Channeling Crystal in your hand and focus on or consider the problem or area that you need help with.

"Listen" carefully but remember that the answer might not come immediately. Often, in the beginning you may find that you wake up some morning and seem to "know" what to do.

When you are working on a problem, keep the Channeling Crystal with you as much as possible and keep it close at night. Sometimes that is the only time the answers can come clearly when you are just starting to open yourself.

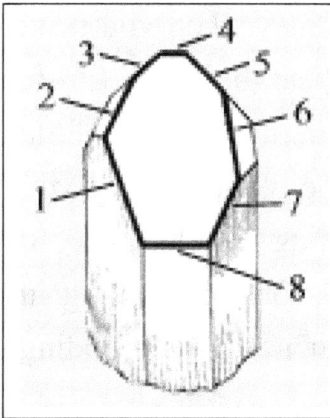

Grounding Crystals have **eight edges** surrounding the largest sloping face. They are quite rare and not always available. Grounding is the ability to deal with practical matters in a realistic way.

For example, in dealing with the question "How am I going to make a living", a grounded person will consider his/her skills and decide how best to use those skills to make a living. An ungrounded or "spacey" person does not like to deal with the practical or realistic aspects of life.

Grounding Crystals help you deal with practical matters in a realistic way. They connect you with the earth and keep your energies from being scattered. They help you think clearly and express yourself clearly.

When used in meditation, they help you form a strong connection with higher knowledge, but keep you grounded so that you can apply the information in practical terms.

When using a Grounding Crystal to work through a personal problem, remember that it will require you to look at the truth of the situation and compel you to deal with the truth.

It is sometimes difficult to recognize times when you need this crystal because not being grounded can be a way of life for some people. These days, it is common to be a little spacey because of things going on in the world. When you are having trouble concentrating, feeling a reluctance to tackle a task that needs doing, or find yourself running in circles but accomplishing nothing, you need a Grounding Crystal.

Exercise

Sit quietly holding the crystal. Visualize yourself firmly rooted to the earth. Breathe deeply and visualize the roots going deeper into the earth. Continue this exercise until you feel calm and peaceful. When you are having a "spacey" time be sure to keep your Grounding Crystal close to you. Some people may need to keep it with them most of the time. You can sometimes help another person become more grounded by sitting quietly, holding your Grounding Crystal, and visualizing that person being firmly rooted to the earth.

Window	Window Crystals have a small diamond shaped face which takes the place of one of the corners where two of the parallel faces usually meet the corresponding two sloping faces.

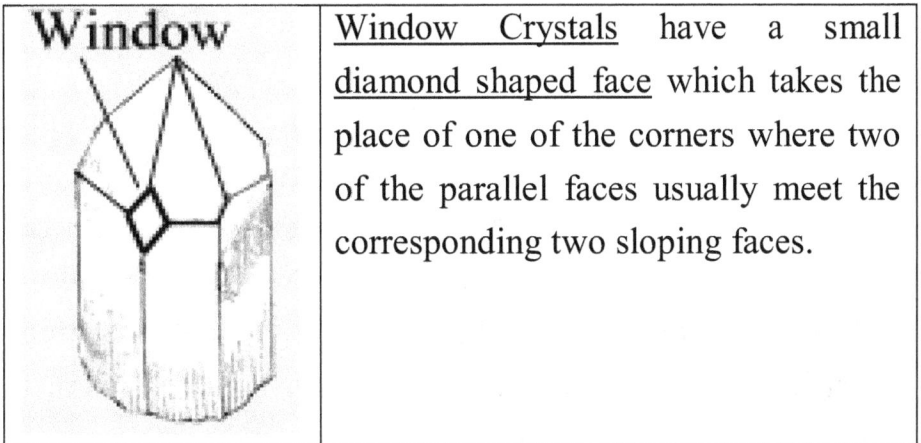

Window Crystals are introspection crystals in that they help you see what is inside yourself. They help bring things to the surface so you can see them and effectively deal with them. If you are having problems and are not sure why, a Window Crystal can be a good help.

Window Crystals are used for working within yourself to deal with problems and changes that must be made in your life. They are used in meditation to help you solve problems that are troubling your Inner Being. For example, if you find you are very jealous of a friend, you can use a Window Crystal to work within yourself to find the reason and deal with it.

Think of a Window Crystal as a window into your soul. These are very personal crystals, and when one comes into your hands, it is intended to help you specifically.

Exercise

Sit with the crystal in your hand and concentrate on whatever there is within you that needs dealing with or changing. Just sit quietly and allow your mind to go where it wants to go. If you are not sure what changes you need to make, sit with the crystal and ask it directly to help you find the areas in your life that may be causing you problems that you are not aware of.

This crystal can be used when trying to help someone else solve problems. If a friend comes to you to talk about a problem have him/her hold the Window Crystal while you talk. It can help him/her open up.

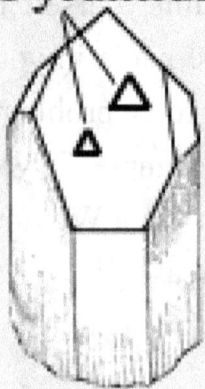

| Pyramids | Record Keepers have a pyramid shaped indention or elevation that appears to be etched on one of the sloping sides. These are fairly rare, and often the pyramid will not be noticed until the crystal comes into the hands of the person it was meant to work with. Sometimes the pyramid can disappear and sometimes more pyramids show up. Each of these crystals has its own special lesson to teach, usually the lesson the person most needs to learn. |

Record Keepers differ from Window Crystals in that Window Crystals help you look inside yourself to let you see the various things you need to learn, while Record Keepers deal with a specific lesson that you need to learn. A Record Keeper will often pass from your hands very quickly once the lesson is learned.

Carry your Record Keeper or put it close to your bed so that it can work with you. It can also be used for meditation.

Some crystals have special characteristics, eg. an Isis with a Record Keeper. In this case, there is a specific lesson to learn that deals with the feminine side of your energy. If you have an Isis with a Window it means that you need to look inside to find the areas in your feminine side that are causing you problems.

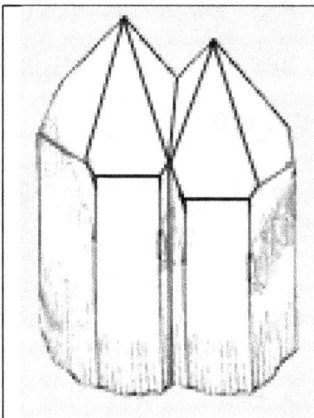

Twin Crystals have two terminations (points) at the same end, which have developed from a single base. You can tell a Twin Crystal from two crystals that are simply attached to each other, by the fact that both parts of a Twin Crystal are exactly parallel to each other, and have no boundary between them in at least a small region of the crystal.

These are wonderful crystals to use when dealing with "relationship" things. They can help you gain insight into the underlying problems in a relationship, and help work through them.

They can generate very positive energy towards improving a relationship. This works for any kind of a relationship, not only a man-woman relationship.

A Twin with a rainbow can be very effectively used to project healing energy into a relationship or to keep a good relationship strong.

When you are having a problem with a relationship, sit quietly with the Twin and ask for help. Remember, the answers come from many directions.

Twins are personal crystals as one of the Twins is very closely tuned to your energy, so it is not possible to use this crystal to work for others in relationship matters.

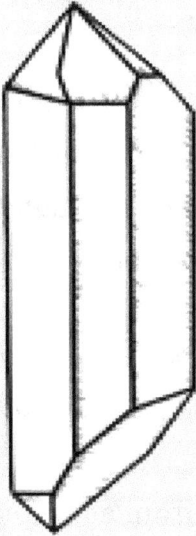

<u>Double Terminated Crystals</u> are crystals that have <u>points at both ends</u>, allowing energy to flow readily in both directions. Double Terminated Crystals strengthen energy flow, and are especially useful when you need to share or exchange energy between you and another person. They are useful when you are working to help other people, for example in massage or counselling, where energy needs to flow in both directions. In these situations, energy flows toward you when you tune into a person to find out what that person needs, and energy flows from you when you give the person needed healing energy. Double Terminated Crystals are very important to people doing healing work for themselves or others. They also help teach sharing through energy exchange.

<u>Exercise</u>

If you are feeling out of balance with the world, sit quietly and hold the Double Terminated Crystal in your right hand. Visualize white light flowing into the first point, through the crystal and out the other point directly into your body.

If working with someone else, visualize energy flowing into you through the top of your head, down your arm, through the crystal, and into the other person. This can be done while you are with the person or it can work from a distance.

If you have children, try using this crystal to send positive energy to the child when the child is upset or angry. It can have a calming effect on both of you.

Rainbow Crystals have a rainbow reflected from within the crystal. Usually they are best viewed in sunlight. These crystals are especially good as meditation crystals for working deep within the subconscious. They work particularly well to lighten the mood for people experiencing sadness, grief or depression. Just holding a Rainbow Crystal can lighten your mood. Rainbow Crystals are also very good at drawing negativity from a room or a situation. Always cleanse a crystal that has been used to clear negativity by letting it sit in the sunshine for a while.

Exercise

Rainbow Crystals bring joy into your life. If you are sad or depressed, sit and meditate on the Rainbow. It can help lighten your mood. If working with another, let him/her hold the crystal if he/she is with you. Otherwise, hold the Rainbow and visualize white light leaving the rainbow and going to him/her.

Baby

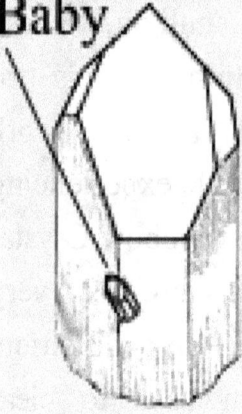

Crystals With Babies are crystals that have tiny crystals growing inside a larger crystal. These are very good for people who have had traumatic childhoods, physically or emotionally. They are helpful for people who are blocking painful memories. They help bring the cause of pain to the surface and allow the person to successfully deal with it, while shielding that person from the pain those memories can cause. These crystals work well for people who are working through current family problems. Work slowly with this type of crystal, so that things can be cleared at your own pace.

You may not feel inclined to work with it at all in the beginning. Do not force yourself. When you are ready, you will find yourself drawn to that particular crystal. You may have this crystal for years before you use it. Also, sometimes crystals come to you so that they can go to someone else.

For example, someone might receive a Crystal With Babies, have it for some time and not be drawn to it at all. Suddenly they have an urge to pass it on to someone else.

You can use this crystal in meditation or just keep it close to you. Just be prepared to deal with whatever comes up. Try to have some support around you if you are going to work with this crystal.

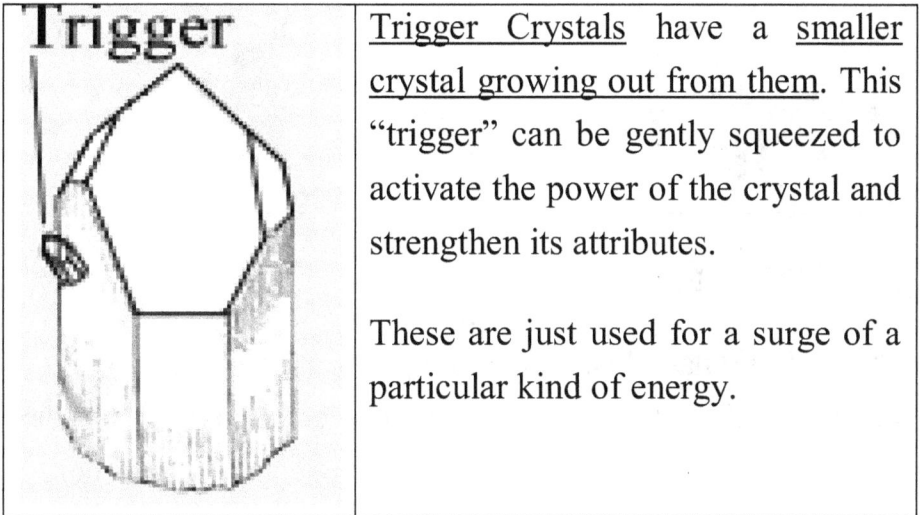

Trigger	Trigger Crystals have a smaller crystal growing out from them. This "trigger" can be gently squeezed to activate the power of the crystal and strengthen its attributes. These are just used for a surge of a particular kind of energy.

A Self Healed Crystal is one that has been broken off and damaged quite badly, but then begins to grow again. A Phantom Crystal is a crystal that has had some impurity drop on it during growth, but then continues to grow right around the impurity.

Each of these types can help you heal from being hurt, can help you heal from emotional injuries. These are important crystals that will usually come into your life at a time when you are carrying a lot of pain. Just sitting with either crystal will help you deal with the pain effectively.

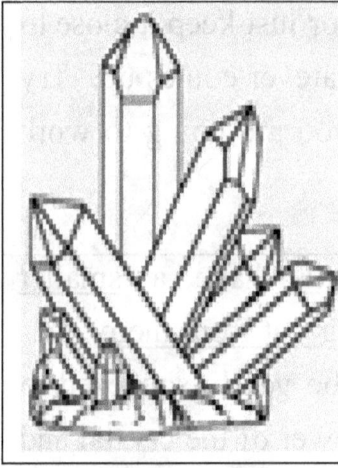

Clusters represent community and are very powerful at clearing any negative energy from a room.

Just set one out somewhere and allow it to work to clear the environment.

Amethyst / Smoky Clusters

These particular clusters are mined in a very small area of the Colorado Rockies. They are powerful in keeping the spirit centered because they carry a special kind of energy that keeps all the energy centers within the body aligned, balanced, and in harmony with each other.

Brazilian Crystals

Crystals from Brazil have the special quality of enhancing your ability to project energy over a distance. For example, in some of the exercises cited herein, where you are sending healing energy to someone that is too far away for you to touch physically, hold a Brazilian crystal along with the other crystal to strengthen the transmission.

Tibetan Crystals

These extremely rare crystals are hand mined high in the mountains of Tibet, and are carried down the mountainside by backpack. Tibetan crystals are for protection. Just having a Tibetan crystal close to you puts up an automatic shield against negative energy. It also helps shield you from other people's negative energy. This shield is even stronger if you do a centering exercise while holding the crystal.

Copyright © John and Micki Baumann [31]

Reprinted with permission.

---

[31] http://www.lovesedona.com/

Earlier cultures understood water much better than we do today. Pure water was treasured. The ancient Chinese saved water in jade vases, Incas and Aztecs in obsidian jars and African witchdoctors used quartz. One thing modern research has now proved, is that the high silica content of all these minerals allows water to keep its structure and prevent it from becoming "weak" and polluted.

Natural water found in many springs, rivers and lakes has its outer electrons complete. This is one of the keys to healthy water: how many electrons the water has or doesn't have. Unstructured water, simply put, is missing one electron from its outer orbit whereas structured water, by comparison, has no missing electrons.

Water can be de-structured not only by the addition of harmful chemicals, but also by its now almost universal transportation. When it moves through pressurized pipes it is forced to move in an artificial way instead of its natural spirals. When water moves through pipes it forces the outer electrons to be removed, creating unstructured water.

This means that all water that we drink or bathe in that comes from pressurized pipes is associated with disease. And when we bathe in water we absorb through our skin sixteen ounces in twenty minutes! It is the same as if we drank the water. Perhaps mankind has now made a similar mistake to the Romans with their use of lead plates and utensils.

Water, the lifeblood of Mother Earth, is much more than hydrogen and oxygen. It is a mysterious, crystalline living entity which nurtures all life on Earth. It is a powerful carrier, mediator and producer of energy. It has the ability to link, transform and carry physical elements and subtle energies. Flower and gem elixirs are a good example of the latter. Over 70% of our bodies and the planet is water. The necessity of healthy, structured water cannot be exaggerated.

A Simple and Inexpensive Way to Safely and Effectively Structure Water

You will need ......

[1] 6 quartz crystal points (single crystals) of any size

[2] 1 double terminated (a point at each end) quartz crystal of any size (optional)

[3] clear glass container (glass or bowl)

[4] The purest water you can find. Don't be discouraged if this is not ideal, we can only work with what we have. The following process will certainly make an improvement to any water.

[5] A clear intention to re-structure and energize the water. Quartz interacts with the human mind, so try this with optimum results.

This is what you will need to do ......

[1] Clean the crystals by holding them under cold running water for a few minutes.

[2] Fill a plain glass bowl with water.

[3] Place the double terminated crystal in the middle of the water.

[4] Arrange the 6 points equally around the container (facing in), to form a hexagon.

[5] Visualize the points charging the DT and the water with vital, healing energy.

[6] Visualize the DT charging the water with vital, healing energy.

Steps 5 and 6 are not essential as quartz crystals will structure the water anyway. However, it does amplify the process and allows the more experienced scope for more precise intentions.

Leave this arrangement where it will be undisturbed for several hours or overnight. If you are leaving it outside, cover with a plain glass sheet to prevent contamination. Drink this water every day. Make fresh daily. Research has shown that even naturally structured spring water loses its energy when placed in sealed containers for over four hours.

The word chakra comes from the ancient Sanskrit word for wheel.

Chakras are specialized centres through which life energy is absorbed and distributed to our cells, organs and body tissues. The integrity of the flow of energy throughout the body system is strongly affected by

[1] our personality

[2] our emotions

[3] what we say

[4] what we think and believe of ourselves

In most of us, this flow is depleted, blocked or compromised, thereby substantially contributing to the lack of well-being that many experience.

While the energetic system contains hundreds of minor chakras, there are 7 major ones.

The first (Root chakra) is located at the base of the spine.

The second (Sacral chakra) is located just below the navel.

The third (Solar Plexus chakra) is located above the pit of the stomach.

The fourth (Heart chakra) is located in the middle of the breastbone.

The fifth (Throat chakra) is located in the area of the throat.

The sixth (Third Eye or Brow chakra) is located between the eyes

The seventh (Crown chakra) is located on the top of the head.

Each of these chakras is associated with a color that follows the rainbow. Starting at the root, we go from red, orange, yellow, green, sky-blue, and indigo, ending with violet at the crown.

Sounds, emotions and organs are also associated with each chakra.

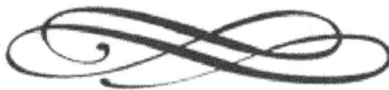

ROOT CHAKRA

Scale Equivalent: Do

Red stones for activating and energizing: Garnet, Ruby, Bloodstone, Jasper (red), Spinel (red).

Black stones for calming and balancing: Smoky Quartz (dark), Tourmaline (black), Apache Tear, Onyx, Jet.

Green stones for toning down or reversing: Aventurine (green), Jade (green), Dioptase, Emerald, Malachite, Tourmaline (green), Chrysoprase, Unakite, Dendritic Agate, Moss Agate, Fluorite (green), Nephrite, Bloodstone.

SACRAL (Belly) CHAKRA

Scale Equivalent: Re

Orange stones for activating: Carnelian, Citrine Quartz (dark), Coral (red), Jacinth, Salmon Jade, Copper, Calcite (orange).

Brown stones for balancing: Jasper (brown), Tiger Eye, Boji Stone, Magnetite (Lodestone), Sardonyx, Chiastolite, Mahogany Obsidian.

Blue stones for toning down or reversing: Chrysocolla, Turquoise, Topaz (blue), Blue Lace Agate, Celestite, Aquamarine, Amazonite, Tourmaline (blue), Larimar.

SOLAR PLEXUS CHAKRA

Scale Equivalent: Mi

Yellow stones for activating: Citrine Quartz (light), Topaz (golden), Amber, Sunstone, Pyrite, Jasper (yellow), Fluorite (yellow), Tourmaline (yellow).

Yellow/green stones for balancing: Peridot.

Violet stones for toning down or reversing: Amethyst, Tourmaline (violet), Fluorite (violet), Sugilite, Alexandrite, Charoite, Tanzanite, Iolite, Lepidolite.

HEART CHAKRA

Scale Equivalent: Fa

Green stones for activating: Aventurine (green), Jade (green), Dioptase, Emerald, Malachite, Tourmaline (green), Chrysoprase, Unakite, Dendritic Agate, Moss Agate, Fluorite (green), Nephrite, Bloodstone.

Pink stones for balancing: Rose Quartz, Kunzite, Tourmaline (pink), Rhodochrosite, Rhodonite, Carnelian (pink), Watermelon Tourmaline, Morganite.

Red stones for toning down or reversing: Garnet, Ruby, Bloodstone, Jasper (red), Spinel (red).

THROAT CHAKRA

Scale Equivalent: So

Blue stones for activating: Chrysocolla, Turquoise, Amazonite, Tourmaline (blue), Larimar.

Aqua stones for balancing: Topaz (blue), Blue Lace Agate, Celestite, Aquamarine.

Orange stones for toning down or reversing: Carnelian, Citrine Quartz (dark), Coral (red), Jacinth, Salmon Jade, Copper, Calcite (orange).

BROW (Third Eye) CHAKRA

Scale Equivalent: La

Indigo Blue stones for activating: Lapis Lazuli, Sodalite, Sapphire, Azurite, Kyanite, Fluorite (blue) Holly Blue Agate, Tourmaline (blue), Jasper (blue).

White stones for balancing: Moonstone, White Agate, Selenite, Opal, Snow Quartz.

Orange stones for toning down or reversing: Carnelian, Citrine Quartz (dark), Coral (red), Jacinth, Salmon Jade, Copper, Calcite (orange).

CROWN CHAKRA

Scale Equivalent: Ti

Violet stones for activating: Amethyst, Tourmaline (violet), Fluorite (violet), Sugilite, Alexandrite, Charoite, Tanzanite, Iolite, Lepidolite.

White stones for balancing: Moonstone, White Agate, Selenite, Opal, Snow Quartz.

Yellow stones for toning down or reversing: Citrine Quartz (light), Topaz, (golden), Amber, Sunstone, Pyrite, Jasper (yellow), Fluorite (yellow), Tourmaline (yellow).

TRANSPERSONAL CHAKRA (above the head)

Scale Equivalent: Do

Clear stones for activating and balancing: Clear Quartz, Diamond, Zircon, Herkimer Diamond, Fluorite (clear), Danburite.

Mini Reiki treatments are basically chakra balancing. There are a number of different ways to do this with a seated client.

The first involves putting your hands on the forehead and back of the head as the first position. Move to the throat and back of the neck next, followed by the heart chakra and hand behind to match. Move to the solar plexus and behind to match, followed by the sacral chakra and hand behind to match. Lastly, the root chakra and hand behind to match. This can also be done from the root chakra and working your way up.

The time spent on each chakra will depend on how "off" they are. Several minutes each are all that is usually required. Once you use these methods and become familiar with the Reiki energy, you will be able to use your own intuition as to how long for each position as well as which method works best for you and your client.

Crystal healing layouts refer to the placement of crystals on or around the body, in a particular pattern, to rejuvenate, refresh or heal the mind and body. It has been said that this ancient art of the laying on of stones dates back to the civilizations of Lemuria and Atlantis.

Crystal healing addresses all levels of our beingness: physical, mental, emotional and spiritual. Crystal layouts can be used to increase the flow of energy, to correct imbalances in the physical and subtle bodies, and to connect with the mineral kingdom in a different and deeper way.

Please refer to the Book Source Bibliography for useful information.

Crystal Healing Layouts [32]

Crystal Grids and Layouts [33]

7 Chakra Crystal Healing Layout [34]

------

[32] http://www.crystalwellbeing.co.uk/crystalhealing/healinglayouts.php
[33] http://www.pebblesspiritualcave.com/CrystalGridsLayouts.html
[34] http://www.reiki-for-holistic-health.com/reiki-healing-with-crystals.html

THE SEAL OF SOLOMON LAYOUT

Referred to as The Seal of Solomon because a six pointed star, formed from two interlocking triangles, was often used in medieval magical texts ascribed to King Solomon. The symbol represents the interaction of the four elements and the uniting of heaven and earth.

The Seal of Solomon can be used whenever there is a need to relax, physically and mentally. It refreshes the body's energies and clears away stress. You will need six clear quartz points, which should be placed in a star shape evenly around the body: at head and feet, at shoulder level and knee level.

When the points are facing outward there will be a release of any excess energy. When the points face toward the body there will be a charging, energizing effect.

Begin with the points turned outwards for about five minutes, then reverse the stones so that the body is infused with new energy for a minute or two. If you experience any discomfort when the stones are facing in the first direction, try starting with the other placement.

GROUNDING LAYOUT

In order to be effective when using crystals for healing, and in order to gain maximum benefit from crystal healing, you need to be centered and grounded.

Grounding is a term that means you are solidly anchored in the present, with a certain inner stillness, a feeling of being secure, in control of yourself and alert. When you lack grounding you will feel nervous, unfocused, agitated and unable to concentrate.

Crystals needed include 2 smoky quartz crystal points.

For a grounding layout, place a smoky quartz crystal point downwards at the base of the throat and a second smoky quartz between the legs or close to the base of the spine, also with its point towards the feet.

This is an excellent way to center and ground your energies in a couple of minutes.

Book Source Bibliography

Healing With Crystals by Pamela Chase and Jonathan Pawlik (ISBN 1564145352)

Healing With Gemstones by Pamela Chase and Jonathan Pawlik (ISBN 1564145476)

Crystal Enchantments: A Complete Guide to Stones and Their Magical Properties by D.J. Conway (ISBN 1580910106)

The Illustrated Guide to Crystals by Judy Hall (ISBN 0806936274)

Pocket Guide to Crystals and Gemstones by Sirona Knight (ISBN 0895949474)

Illustrated Elements of Crystal Healing by Simon Lilly (ISBN 0007133871)

Crystal Healing by Sue Lilly and Simon Lilly (ISBN 075480867X)

Crystals and Crystal Healing by Simon Lilly (ISBN 1842153730)

Crystal Decoder by Sue Lilly (ISBN 0764117351)

Healing With Gemstones and Crystals by Diane Stein (ISBN 0895948311)

The Book of Crystal Healing by Liz Simpson (ISBN 0806904178)

Psychic Healing With Spirit Guides and Angels by Diane Stein (Chapter 8) (ISBN 0895948079)

Love Is In The Earth: A Kaleidoscope of Crystals by Melody (ISBN 0962819034)

The Magical Crystal: Expanding Your Crystal Consciousness by Geoffrey Keyte (ISBN 0852072694)

Gemstones and Crystals Book List [35] is a list of resource material that I have compiled on my personal website whereby you can link directly to purchase online.

Pendulum and Dowsing Book List [36] is a list of resource material that I have compiled on my personal website whereby you can link directly to purchase online.

---

[35] http://www.portalsofspirit.com/BooksAboutGems.htm
[36] http://www.portalsofspirit.com/Dowsing.htm

Arkansas Crystal Works [37] (Genn Waite)

Avalon Crystals [38] (Kellie Jo Conn, crystal formations pictures)

Clear Creek Crystal Mine [39] (Stuart Schmitt)

Heaven and Earth Jewelry [40]

Metaphysical and Mystical Healing Properties [41]

Metaphysical Properties Glossary [42]

Metaphysical Properties of Crystals [43]

Metaphysical Properties of Quartz Crystals [44]

---

[37] http://www.arkansascrystalworks.com/
[38] http://www.neatstuff.net/avalon/
[39] http://www.arcrystalmine.com/index.php
[40] http://heavenandearthjewelry.com/
[41] http://crystalsandjewelry.com/metaphysicalproperties.html
[42] http://www.thatcrystalsite.com/guide/properties-glossary.php
[43] http://www.kacha-stones.com/properties_other_crystals.htm
[44] http://www.kacha-stones.com/quartz_crystals_properties.htm

Portals of Spirit: Chakra links [45] (my personal website)

Portals of Spirit: Crystal Links [46] (my personal website)

Portals of Spirit: Gemstone Links [47] (my personal website)

The Crystal Tiger Homepage [48] (Karen Ryan, Crystal Energy Therapist)

The Crystal Tarot: Center for Self-Healing and Empowerment [49]

Therapeutic Gemstones for Healing and Awakening [50]

---

[45] http://www.portalsofspirit.com/chakra.htm
[46] http://www.portalsofspirit.com/crystals.htm
[47] http://www.portalsofspirit.com/gems.htm
[48] http://www.crystaltiger.com/
[49] http://www.thecrystaltarot.com/
[50] http://www.gemisphere.com/gemstones/therapeutic_gemstones.htm

Alternative Healing Academy: Color, Crystal Therapy Practitioner Home Study Course [51]

Alternative Healing Academy: Advanced Color, Crystal Aromatherapy Practitioner Home Study Course [52]

Alternative Healing Academy: Advanced Color, Crystal, Reflexology Practitioner Home Study Course [53]

Atlantis College of Crystal, Reiki and Sound Healing: Crystal and Sound Healing Certified Correspondence Course [54]

The International Academy of Vibrational Therapies: Correspondence and Distance Learning Crystal Therapy [55]

---

[51] http://www.alternativehealingacademy.org/products/details/16/Color-Crystal-Therapy-Practitioner-Home-Study-Course
[52] http://www.alternativehealingacademy.org/products/details/153/Advanced-Color-Crystal-Aromatherapy-Practitioner
[53] http://www.alternativehealingacademy.org/products/details/18/Color-Crystal-Reflexology-Practitioner-Home-Study-Course
[54] http://www.atlantiscrystalhealing.com/crystal_course.htm
[55] http://www.crystal-healing.com/correspondence.htm

School of Natural Health Sciences: Crystal Healing Home Study Diploma Course [56]

Stonebridge Associated Colleges (UK): Crystal Healing Practitioner (the course that I completed) [57]

The Crystal Academy of Advanced Healing Arts: Crystal Healing Certification Courses [58]

Vantol College of Crystal Therapy [59]

---

[56] http://www.naturalhealthcourses.com/crystal_healing.htm
[57] https://www.stonebridge.uk.com/course/crystal-healing-practitioner
[58] http://webcrystalacademy.com/Courses.html
[59] http://www.crystalcollege.com/

About the Author

Michele Doucette is webmistress of *Portals of Spirit*, a spirituality website whereby one will find links to (1) *The Enlightened Scribe*, (2) an ezine called *Gateway To The Soul*, (3) books of spiritual resonance as well as authors of metaphysical importance, (4) categories of interest from Angels to Zen, (5) up-to-date information as shared by a Quantum Healer, (6) affiliate programs and resources of personal significance, (7) healing resource advertisements and (8) spiritual news.

As a Level 2 Reiki Practitioner, she sends long distance Reiki to those who make the request, claiming only to be a *facilitator of the Universal Energy*, meaning that it is up to the individual(s) in question to use these energies in order to heal themselves.

Having also acquired a Crystal Healing Practitioner diploma (Stonebridge College in the UK), she is guardian to many from the mineral kingdom.

The author of several other spiritual/metaphysical tomes; namely, *The Ultimate Enlightenment For 2012: All We Need Is Ourselves*, *Turn Off The TV: Turn On Your Mind*, *Veracity At Its Best* and *The Collective: Essays on Reality*, all of which have been released as paperback editions through St. Clair Publications.

In addition, she has also written *A Travel in Time to Grand Pré*, a visionary metaphysical title that historically ties the descendants of Yeshua to modern day Nova Scotia.

Against the backdrop of 1754 Acadie, it was the blending of French Acadian history with current DNA testing that allowed for the weaving of this alchemical tale of time travel, romance and intrigue.

From Henry I Sinclair to the Merovingians, from the Cathari treasure at Montségur to the Knights Templar, this novel, together with the words of Yeshua as spoken at the height of his ministry, has the potential to inspire others; for it is herein that we learn how individuals can find their way, their truth(s), so as to live their lives to the fullest.

www.ingramcontent.com/pod-product-compliance
Lightning Source LLC
Chambersburg PA
CBHW060852280326
41934CB00007B/1022